NEEDS NO WORDS

The adoption story of a teen with cancer

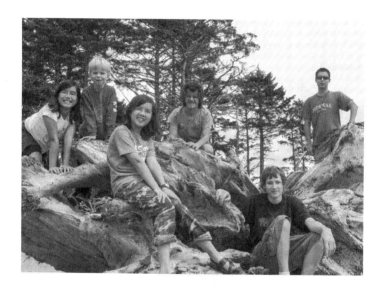

CINDY LOCKE

Cindy Locke

Copyright © 2013 by Cindy Locke

ISBN-13:
978-1492923206

ISBN-10:
1492923206

DEDICATION

My husband Lenny, thank you for embracing my dream of parenting Ivan along with all the other kids that we have parented together over the years. Thank you for taking over my duties along with your own when Ivan became ill.

My children Emily, Jordan, Sarah, Kailey, and Josiah- You loved Ivan as a brother and accepted him into your heart as if he had always been a part of this family. You hurt along with me as he struggled with the cancer. I am so proud to call you my children.

Seneca, thank you for sharing Ivan with us and embracing our family. You truly have become part of our family, even without the blood lines or paperwork to make it official

My son Ivan, thank you for loving me and bringing such joy to my life. I will never be the same. You left an imprint and a legacy for us all.

Cindy Locke

CONTENTS

CONTENTS _____v

ACKNOWLEDGMENTS_____vii

INTRODUCTION _____ix

CHAPTER 1 _____1

CHAPTER 2 _____29

CHAPTER 3 _____51

CHAPTER 4 _____81

CHAPTER 5 _____93

CHAPTER 6 _____113

CHAPTER 7 _____135

CHAPTER 8 _____145

CHAPTER 9 _____153

CHAPTER 10 _____181

ACKNOWLEDGMENTS

To Debbie Onishi, Sarah Brouwer, Susan Emery, Grace Bartlett, and especially Alisa Roebke, thank you for the hours you spent assisting in the editing. I had a story to tell but grammar and punctuation was never a strength of mine.

To my daughter and biggest cheerleader, Sarah Locke, thank you for always encouraging me to keep going when I wanted to stop and for helping me with the content and editing.

To Seneca, thank you for allowing me to share some of your personal life with the readers. I could not have told Ivan's story without telling yours.

To my many friends and family, thank you for investing into Ivan's life and encouraging me to tell his story.

Cindy Locke

INTRODUCTION

As a young nurse working on the rehabilitation unit at Seattle Children's Hospital, I provided specialized care to children dealing with a wide variety of medical and social situations. Many were well loved and had great support systems. These kids were never left without at least one family member staying with them at any given moment of the night or day. These children had parents or grandparents, or aunts and uncles that would sleep in uncomfortable chairs in noisy rooms so that their beloved child would never feel alone.

Other children were happy to have one visitor a week for a couple of hours. Some went weeks without any family members by their bedsides. These kids that we cared for faced the most difficult and frightening time in their lives. They dealt with paralysis from spinal cord injuries, traumatic brain injuries, burns, cancer and other life changing and life threatening conditions. These kids needed family. They needed more emotional support than the nursing staff was able to provide them.

As a nurse, there is a limit to the amount of emotional support that one can give a patient. At times, I just wanted to sit and hold a frightened or hurt child. However, my role was nurse, not mother. The amount of care my heart desired to give these children, especially the "motherless" ones, was not practical or appropriate for my role as a nurse.

During my drive home one evening, I poured out my sadness and frustration to God. "I love these kids." "I hurt for these kids." As I reached my home I pulled my little blue station wagon into my driveway. I sat there for a couple minutes just thinking over the situation of my little patients. As I prayed, I began to weep uncontrollably as I heard the spirit of God saying, "You think you hurt for these kids? Feel this." I had to lay the driver's seat back as the waves of grief and emotional pain shook my body. In that moment, I believe that I had actually felt the heart of God. His love and hurt for these children was so raw. In that moment the course of my life was changed forever. Over the next 25 years, hurting children became part of my daily life as my roles changed from nurse to mom.

THE HEART

NEEDS NO WORDS

Cindy Locke

CHAPTER 1

We were a patchwork household of eight. My husband Lenny entered my life as the medical supply and oxygen delivery man to my three medically fragile foster kids. I was in my mid-twenties then and he thought I was just a nurse who worked at the home. I remember his surprise when he realized the house was mine and the three kids were my foster children. To him, this didn't matter and he asked me out on a date. By the second date we'd decided that neither of us enjoyed dating, so after a long day trip, we decided to skip the awkward dating phase and just get married. Before I agreed, I told him that I came as a package deal; me, the kids and the dream. He said "yes" to all of us. Four months after our first date, we said our vows surrounded by friends and family. With that, Lenny and I began our journey of loving the kids that came into our lives. The circumstances may not have been entirely typical, but I knew in my heart, he was the kind of man I wanted in my life and the lives of my children.

I gave birth to our son Jordan eleven months after Lenny and I married, making him our first "homemade" child. Jordan is a very fact based person with very little artistic interest or abilities. He tends to be reserved and quiet.

Emily, four months older than Jordan, joined our family at the age of 2. She was born with a rare syndrome which caused dwarfism, developmental delays, as well as different skeletal abnormalities. She was tiny and frail but we immediately loved her sense of humor and spirit. We finalized her adoption when she was 3 years old. To this day Emily continues to be creative, artistic, and outgoing. Compared to Jordan's personality, Emily is the polar opposite. Raising the two of them was like raising twins.

Our next two kids were "homemade." Sarah and

Kailey are twenty months apart, with Sarah being the oldest. They've almost always shared a room together, and are each other's best friend and constant companion. Both girls have kind and gentle hearts.

Our youngest, Josiah, joined our family as a foster child when he was almost two years old. We adopted him at the age of four when parental rights were terminated. Our blond haired, blue eyed boy had been labeled failure to thrive, was skeletal thin, and extremely fearful when he came to us. He is still small in frame but healthy and happy.

My Grandma Rose had been living with us for several years after she and my Grandpa Chester realized that they could no longer live independently because of their failing health. Grandma was legally blind and walked with a walker. She was still able to get around and take care of most her needs by herself. Our five kids loved to spend time with her in her little studio apartment in the back of our house. She had plenty of time to sit and listen to their stories and she always had cookies or candies on hand to share with them. My Grandparents had been a powerful influence on my life as a young girl and consistently demonstrated how people of faith loved and lived.

I remember one time when I was about 12 years old; my grandfather had taken me to the Greyhound bus station to travel home. While we sat there we noticed a woman who was alone struggling to carry her bags and packages. As everyone looked on or tried to ignore her, my Grandfather raced to her aid. Perhaps a little thing, but to my young mind it was profound. His examples taught me, that if someone is in need and you have the ability to help, the right thing to do is help. At the age of 93, four months after moving in with our family, Grandpa Chester passed away. It was an honor to care for him in his final days.

After our marriage, Lenny and I continued the dream, and kept our house open as a placement for foster children. We experienced the joys and sorrows of foster care as a family, with some placements being better suited for us than others. Some placements became adoptions, as in the case of Josiah and Emily, where others taught us how to let go. Foster care was not always fun and games, it was hard work. Parenting in general is not always easy, but parenting children who are already "half-raised" can be even more difficult.

One of our most traumatizing cases came from our 12 year old foster son Paul (not his real name). He became violent towards me, and though he was young, he was still strong enough to overpower me and leave bruising. We had cautiously taken Paul with the intent to adopt him only after we had been assured that he had no violent tendencies or sexual acting out behaviors. Shortly after he moved into our home he began sharing with my father how he didn't feel that women and girls were as important as men and boys. They were on the hierarchy a little higher than animals, but not even quite human. That was very troubling to both my father and me. I wondered where he had picked up that viewpoint and how deeply it was ingrained in him.

He had been with our family three months when he began violently attacking me with little or no warning. The first time happened while the other children watched and Jordan, 11 years old at the time, tried to protect me. The second and last time he attacked me was even more violent than the first. Outraged over what he was to eat for lunch he punched me with all his might in the chest yelling with wild eyes, "I'm going to kill you." As he continued to scream, I ran to the other room and called 911. I was shaking and stunned by the whole assault. I had never been attacked like that in my life. I had never even witnessed that sort of violence except on TV. Within minutes a sheriff arrived to arrest Paul, taking him to juvenile detention. I noticed as he left in handcuffs that he was beginning to grow a large bump on his forehead. I found out later that he had taken a glass canning jar and smashed it on his own forehead. Thankfully the other kids were at the other end of the house and did not have to witness the assault.

The next day Lenny and I were asked to pick him up from juvenile detention. He seemed bubbly and happy when we arrived, but not because we were there to retrieve him. Instead, he was excited to show off his jail clothes. He was enamored with how he looked in his orange jumpsuit. After he was released to us, we had a long quiet drive home. We waited until we arrived at our house to tell him that his caseworker was on her way to pick him up. He should have known what was going to happen, as we had written a behavioral contract with him after the first incident. It clearly stated if he assaulted a family member again, it would be cause for a removal from our family and we would not proceed with the adoption. He may have signed the contract but he didn't believe that it would actually happen. Even though he had only been with us a relatively short time we had already began to feel like we were his parents. We wanted the best for him, to be the ones to help change the course of his life, and to love him in good times and bad. Unfortunately this was not meant to be, and though it pained us greatly, we knew we could not adequately give Paul the care he needed while still protecting our other vulnerable children.

Paul was stunned and grief stricken at the thought of leaving. He cried and I held him. The boy that sat next to me then was not the same boy that had attacked me 24 hours earlier. Later that afternoon his caseworker came, we loaded his belongings into her car and they drove away. We never saw him again and have no idea what has become of his life.

We were told after the attack that Paul had been violent in other homes and removed. It had been a few months since his last outburst, so the caseworker felt she did not need to share that information with us prior to placement. I believe the goal was to get Paul adopted, if the whole truth was revealed it was unlikely that a family would be found. Even with that information I felt ashamed that I had failed him; that I had abandoned him. I grieved for him and worried about what might become of his life. I wrestled between knowing that he was entering the teen years with more strength and the potential for increased violence, and wanting to influence his life and help turn him in a different direction. No matter how much I rationalized that for the safety of our family Paul had to leave, emotionally I was traumatized by the event. I realized just how risky and difficult foster care could be. Lenny and I began to reconsider continuing foster parenting.

We were already signed up to go on a mission trip to Mexico with Jordan and Emily prior to this happening. The mission trip was a nine day adventure with a group of 6th graders and their parents from our church. We stayed at an orphanage and helped with construction projects and ran a soccer clinic in a nearby village. We spent meals and free time interacting and playing with the kids from the orphanage. One evening, mid-way through our trip, Lenny and I walked up on a little moonlit hill. We talked about all we were experiencing on this trip. Seeing all the beautiful children that had no parents was heart breaking. We knew that we could not stop caring for and loving hurt children. We would continue to be foster parents, but we decided that older boys were too much of a risk for our young family.

Our experiences doing foster care shaped the way we raised our family. We did our best to protect, love, and teach our children how to be kind. One warm August morning, my Grandma Rose was busy going about her morning routine in her little studio apartment. Our 5 kids were home with me just hanging out and enjoying the freedom that summer vacation brings. Josiah, 6 years old, was out catching bugs, his favorite past time in the summer. He loved catching different types of ants and putting them together to see what would happen.

I was scheduled to bring cookies to a meeting I was attending that evening. I had recruited Jordan, then age 16, to help me make several batches for the event. He, more than the rest of the kids, seemed to enjoy baking and excelled in the kitchen. While Jordan added the ingredients, I snuck off to do a quick check of my e-mail. Upon opening one of my emails I saw the subject line "*15 yo boy from Alaska recovering from cancer needs home.*" My caseworker, Darby, from our private foster/adoption agency had forwarded it to me with a note saying, "*I don't know the situation with your friend's child, but thought of you for this young man if you are open and available?*" My world seemed to stop momentarily as I tried to process this e-mail.

The friends that she was referring to were our dear friends, John and Susan. In January of the same year their three month old son, Brent, had nearly died as a result of an undiagnosed liver tumor that had ruptured. He had spent over forty days in intensive care, barely clinging to life. He then spent several more months in and out of the oncology unit. Brent had just finished up chemotherapy a couple months prior when this email arrived in my inbox. This family had become our "God assignment" during those terrifying months. Our focus over that year had been to come alongside and support our friends as their family life had been turned upside down by Brent's cancer. Our two families had become like one big family during those months. John and Susan had four children, Stephanie age 13, Robyn age 11, and John Jay age 9, along with little Brent. On top of all this, their son John Jay has autism. I had recently begun providing occasional respite care for John Jay at our home to give him a break from being around his baby brother. Brent's crying was causing a sensory overload for John Jay. He was having major meltdowns during the summer when he had to endure the baby's cries; not having the benefit of getting away from the noise during the school day. Our family had come to love all the kids in this family; I especially had a heart for John Jay. We had walked closely with John and Susan through all the pain and suffering that cancer brings to the patient and the family. Now I was getting an e-mail asking if we wanted to go down that road ourselves.

I opened the attachment that accompanied Darby's letter. It read,

"Good Morning! This is an unusual request, and I am hoping that there is a home out there to help this boy--- Ivan is a 15 year old Native (Alaskan Native) and Caucasian boy who is currently at Children's Hospital undergoing treatment for cancer. He is a dependent of Alaska State. His older (adult) brother relocated to try and help care for him, and the plan is to eventually place with the older brother, but he needs time to find a job and a home. The request is for a home for 6-9 months,

until the older brother can take him in. Ivan will need to continue treatment via Children's Hospital after discharge. Other than his battle against cancer, he's a 'normal' teen, who usually follows the rules, doesn't have problems with arguing or related issues. He loves music, video games, computers, skateboarding and snowboarding. He has a great sense of humor, is mellow and "easy to get along with." There are no visits/contact with parents, but he will have phone contact with grandparents and unsupervised visits with brother. Please let me know if you have a home for this youth, thanks!!"

This e-mail was sent by the Alaska Placement Coordinator to over 100 people, mainly caseworkers from state and private foster care agencies.

One and a half years prior, after Josiah's adoption, Lenny and I had decided to take a break from foster care. I had been doing foster care for nearly twenty years and Lenny had been involved 18 of those years. Over that time we only had short breaks between foster children. We had parented around 20 kids long term and had countless others for short term placements. With five busy kids and my Grandmother at home we had decided that it was time for a rest. We always knew that we would return to fostering, but had imagined it might be a couple more years. There was something about that email that compelled me to say "yes" despite the break our family was taking and our last experience with an older boy.

Jordan continued making cookies as I sat at the desk in the rec. room filled with excitement. My passion to help woke up again and I wanted this boy in our home. I quickly dialed Lenny's work number.

"Did you see the e-mail from Darby?" I asked him.

"Yes, I did." Without hesitation he said "Go ahead and call her."

This longing brought me back to the initial surge of overwhelming sorrow that I felt in my car 20 years earlier. That glimpse into the heart of God stayed with me all these years later and I longed to put it in practice once again. I knew that the call to Darby was to get more information about this teen named Ivan, but in my heart he was already our new foster son. I made my next call to Darby.

"Yes, we want to find out about the boy you mentioned in your email". Darby assured me she would try to find out more information from his caseworker and get back to me as soon as she heard anything.

I tried to return to the kitchen to assist Jordan with the cookies, but could not stop thinking about this unknown kid named Ivan. I told Jordan about the e-mail and the little bit I knew about the boy that we were interested in fostering. He was neutral on the whole idea, as he is with most ideas, and just kept on with the chore of baking. I knew however, that if we took this boy it would have a profound impact on Jordan, since they were close in age. Whether the impact would be positive or negative remained to be seen.

My mind did mental gymnastics as I tried to clean up the kitchen. What kind of cancer does he have? What is his prognosis? Does he want to go into foster care or is this a repulsive thought to him? Where are his parents? What does he look like? My friend Susan is half Native Alaskan; will he look like her with the dark black hair, dark eyes, and olive complexion? I realized that he probably had no hair at this time because of the chemo, but wondered what he would look like when his hair grew back. What is his personality like? How disabled is he from the cancer? How much nursing care will he require?

I remembered our friend's infant son, Brent, when he was first discharged from the hospital. His care was so overwhelming to his weary parents. Brent was discharged with a nasogastric tube (NG tube) along with a feeding pump and a Hickman line. A Hickman line is a semi-permanent IV catheter placed in his chest to provide a way to give medication, usually chemotherapy, and draw blood without having to poke him each time. Brent also had multiple meds that were given around the clock. Besides that he had to be monitored constantly for fever, urine output, and other signs of illness. The first time John and Susan brought him home they were so overwhelmed that they admitted him back into the hospital the next day. A few days later, when he was discharged again, Susan and Brent came and stayed at our house. Brent needed around the clock care by at least two people, one to sleep and one to care for him. John was home sick and unable to do half the load until he recovered. Susan and I, working together, were still completely exhausted by the ordeal. Was it going to be that exhausting with Ivan? I also thought about the complications of bringing an unknown teenage boy into our family with three vulnerable daughters and a six year old son. Our family had already been traumatized by Paul. Our children's safety had been put at risk, could we do that again? If he wasn't weakened by the cancer was I going to have problems keeping everyone safe?

So, as these thoughts raced through my mind I continued to go back to the reality that there was some boy suffering with cancer at Children's Hospital without the love of parents. I also wondered about his brother. I knew that John and Susan barely made it through Brent's ordeal, and they had family and friends supporting them the entire way. My heart went out to his brother as well. I knew it must be very difficult to relocate to a different state to care for a family member.

Later that day Darby called and told me that she had forwarded our home study to Ivan's caseworker. A home study is a report describing the family and environment that is available. I was hopeful Darby would receive some sort of information quickly, or that I would receive a call from the caseworker. I had seen the huge list of e-mail addresses that received this letter.

Maybe someone else would want him and we won't even get a chance at bringing him into our family. I was also concerned that the caseworker would think, "YIKES, this family already has five kids and an elderly Grandmother in their care." The caseworker could justifiably think it would be too much for us to take care of a teenager with cancer along with what we already had going.

We didn't hear anything and had to go through the weekend with all the questions unanswered. The following Monday, my 21 year old cousin, flew in from Missouri to spend 11 days with us. She'd spent most of her summer and winter vacations with us since she'd graduated from high school. She was going to college in her home state of Missouri, scheduled to graduate in December. Her plan was to live with us after graduation while she waited for acceptance into a graduate program. Our plan was to paint and decorate the room that would be hers while she was here this summer. We were also planning on going camping at our favorite spot-Hurricane Ridge on the Olympic Peninsula. Monday I was busy getting my cousin from the airport and catching up on the events in her life. Tuesday we painted the room that she would stay in after her graduation. I was happy to have the diversion, but my mind kept going back to wondering about Ivan. I craved more information.

Wednesday I finally received the phone call that I had been waiting on for 6 days. Ivan's caseworker from Alaska, Jami, called to speak with me. I learned that Ivan had Ewing's Sarcoma, which is a type of bone cancer. He had been going through cancer treatment for almost exactly one year. When Ivan's cancer was diagnosed, it had already gone to his lungs. Ivan's cancer treatment was very difficult on him and had already included surgery, chemotherapy, and radiation. Ivan's initial problem was pain in his back which eventually led to paralysis of his legs. His treatment and determination gave him back the strength to walk short distances, and he used a wheelchair for long distance. His brother, Seneca, had been his caregiver the entire time and they had been living at a Ronald McDonald House near the hospital except when Ivan was inpatient. Ivan would be having his end of treatment scans on September 1st, and would be ready to be discharged after they were completed. I also learned that Ivan had spent the past several years in residential treatment centers in Alaska and Montana prior to becoming ill. I was told that he had made good progress while in treatment. Besides being quiet and shy, his behaviors were pretty typical for a teenager at this point.

With all we had been through with Paul, I still believed this caseworker was honest when she told me this teen was stable enough emotionally to be placed in a family. She also told me that besides us, only one other person had responded to the e-mail and the other person was not a licensed foster home but they were a native family. I assured her that we felt confident that we could care well for Ivan. With my nursing background, I felt I could handle his medical care. My very close friend Susan was half Native Alaskan like Ivan, and she would surely be available for him if they were concerned about him staying tied to his Native Alaskan culture. I just wanted to yell "Please pick us!" His social worker, Jami, said that she would let us know if our family was chosen.

After the phone call I was incredibly excited. I knew that it wasn't official, but I felt pretty confident that we were going to be the family for Ivan. Every time we knew we are receiving a new foster child, I would go into a nesting mode just like when I was pregnant with our three biological children. I start rearranging furniture, decorating their room, buying their clothes, and getting everything I think they might need. The only problem this time is that the best room for Ivan was the room we had just painted for my cousin. It had the bigger closet and I knew he would probably need this space to store all his medical supplies along with all his regular teenager gear. My cousin was so gracious when I asked if she'd mind staying in a different bedroom with the smaller wardrobe closet instead of the room we'd just painted. We were blessed with a large seven bedroom house. The kids were accustomed to shifting around to different rooms in order to accommodate the children and adults that we often had staying with us. So shuffling rooms again wasn't a problem.

Jordan was also going to have to bunk up again with his six year old little brother, Josiah. Jordan was always a good sport about doing this sort of thing. He'd been sharing his room off and on with his little brother for several years. Fortunately, Jordan is a minimalist. He does not collect or need many material items. He actually has very few possessions and his room is quite bare. As long as he has a place to put his computer, do his homework and store his clothes, "he's good". Jordan has called nearly each of the seven bedrooms in our house his room at one time or another. Maybe that is why he has so few belongings. It is just too hard to drag everything around when he's asked to move to a different room to make space for another child.

Our family was able to go camping at Hurricane Ridge. We enjoyed our time together with hikes, campfires, and watching the deer run around the meadows. Amidst the fun, my mind was never diverted for long from thinking about Ivan.

By the next week, mid- August, we learned that our home was chosen and that we should expect his discharge during the first week of September. I was thrilled. I couldn't wait to finally meet him and his brother. Ivan's case worker, Jami gave me the phone number to their room at the Ronald McDonald house. I got to hear Ivan's voice when I called and reached the answering machine. He sounded so young and timid. Later, his older brother Seneca returned my call. I was able to ask him some more questions about Ivan's day to day routine and care needs. Seneca, like Ivan, was very quiet when you first talked with him. He had a slow way of speaking on the phone with long pauses. We were able to set up a time that I could meet both of them the following week. I would have preferred to drive down right that minute, but I didn't want to appear too pushy. Instead I turned my energy into researching his type of cancer and getting everything ready for him.

I began to run Ewing's Sarcoma through the search engine in my computer to read all that I could find on that type of cancer. What I found was terrifying. Since Ivan's cancer had already spread to his lungs when he was diagnosed, his chance of survival was only around 20%, and if his cancer relapsed he virtually had no chance of survival.

As I researched, I remembered hearing about a local teenager that was in the news who also had some sort of cancer. His name was Travis and his story touched me deeply. He just graduated from high school and had given the commencement speech at the ceremony. I remember him saying that he would not be going to college or planning for his future because he only had six months to live. I wondered if by any chance he and Ivan had the same cancer. I searched again on my trusty search engine and found the story. I was shocked; he also had Ewing's Sarcoma. As I re-read the story about this amazing young man, who was so matter- of - fact about facing his own death, I couldn't help but wonder about Ivan's future. I believe in miracles. I had watched little Brent teeter on the brink of death for so long with not much hope of survival and then come back to health. We would just have to start praying that Ivan would also beat the odds.

With this information tucked away inside me, I decided that I wanted to make the most comfortable room for Ivan that I could manage. I ran around to different stores looking for just the right bedding to place on his full size bed. I figured that he would still hang out in or on his bed a lot, so I wanted it to be very comfortable. It also needed to be something a 15 year old boy would like. I chose a really soft light brown bedspread with two body pillows, one dark brown and the other navy blue and brown plaid, along with another brown regular pillow. I placed a small desk next to his bed with a desk lamp and a recliner in the corner of the room. He would also have a book shelf and a large dresser. I wondered if this room wouldn't be just the room he recovered in, but possibly the room he died in. The plan was for him to live with us for six to nine months. I knew that you could never count on the timeline given to you since plans often change. What if Ivan's cancer came back in those 6-9 months? Could his brother take care of him as he was dying, along with working full time?

Death was something our family had dealt with before. I had taken care of my 93 year old Grandfather and a good friend who died of breast cancer. I knew that it was a 24 hour/a day job and it took several people to adequately care for someone who was dying. In many ways my grandfather's life and death challenged me and prepared me to take on caring for Ivan. Ivan was in need of help and I was able to help him through this rough time. Like my Grandfather, I could not turn my back. If the statistics were true and the cancer was to return, my Grandfather had taught me how to care for someone who was dying.

Now Ivan's room was ready for him and so were we. I took a bunch of pictures throughout the house, inside and out. I also took pictures of each family member. We printed these pictures out and labeled everything so Ivan could get an idea of what our family was like. I put all of these in a folder, readying them to be seen when I took them down to show Ivan and Seneca. I wanted him to know who he'd be living with and what the house looked like. The following Monday at 6pm was the time I was going to finally meet the two brothers.

Monday afternoon I received a phone call from Seneca. Our meeting was going to have to be postponed. Ivan had developed a serious infection and was being admitted to ICU because his blood pressure had become unstable. I was devastated. Not only did I desperately want to meet him, but I also wanted to be a support to him while he was sick. I'd have to wait until he was feeling good enough to meet someone new. Thankfully, Seneca agreed to meet me so that I could give him the photos that I had been working on for Ivan.

That evening I was nervous as I prepared to meet Seneca. I had no idea what he looked like as I entered the Ronald McDonald house. I asked at the front desk if they knew where I could find Seneca. They pointed to a young man standing across the room. I don't know what I was thinking he would look like but he was not at all what I had imagined. He was close to six feet tall with impressively large shoulders and arms. He had long shoulder length black hair, and multiple tattoos along with several facial piercings. I was almost afraid to go and speak with him. From a distance, he looked tough and intimidating. I approached him and introduced myself. As I spoke with him I noticed how soft spoken he was. I believe you can tell a lot about a person by their eyes and Seneca had the most gentle eyes. After speaking with him for just a few minutes I was no longer intimidated by his exterior. I could tell he was a gentle soul. We talked about how Ivan was doing with his current infection. I asked Seneca how he was coping with everything. Seneca was very tired. He had been up a lot with Ivan while he was coming down with this new infection. He was also emotionally drained. Ivan was quite angry with him for insisting that he go to the hospital to have this infection checked, which led to his admission.

I was so impressed by the devotion of this older brother. How many brothers would give up everything, move to another state, and care for their younger sibling? Seneca was 7 years older than Ivan. They had lived together until Ivan was 10 and Seneca was 17 years old. Just before Ivan was placed in psychiatric facilities and residential treatments centers, Seneca was also forced to leave the family. He had tried to remain in contact with Ivan but was prevented from doing so. The first time Seneca was able to have contact with Ivan was over four years after they'd been separated. Jami had reached him with the news that his brother was hospitalized with cancer. Ivan, who had gone from a little child to a teenager in those years, was being airlifted to Washington State for treatment. With only a couple days warning Seneca was forced to make the decision to become his brother's caregiver, quit his job, pack what he could take with him, and move to another state. The brothers were nearly strangers to each other after their long separation.

With virtually no other family support, the two of them had gone through a very difficult year filled with chemo, radiation, therapies, illness, and multiple admissions to the hospital including trips to intensive care. Ivan had battled the cancer and Seneca had, with the exception of the hospital staff, single handedly cared for him every step of the way. I shared how impressed I was that he was sacrificing himself to take care of Ivan. I made a promise to Seneca on that first meeting that I would not come between them or keep them apart from one another. I knew they had forged a special bond and I did not want to do anything to harm that. I gave Seneca the folder with the pictures of our home and family and asked him to pass it on to Ivan. When I stood to leave I reached out to give him a hug and he hugged me back for a long time. I could tell that Seneca had suffered a great deal of pain and weariness over the past years, just as I had been told Ivan had.

As I drove home from that meeting I prayed and wondered. What role was I supposed to play in Seneca's life? I was going to be Ivan's foster mom not Seneca's. How was this all going to unfold? From that first meeting Seneca had left an impression on my heart. I left not only caring for Ivan but for his brother as well.

CHAPTER 2

From what little information I had about Ivan's current medical condition, I was worried. I knew he had an infection and his blood pressure was unstable enough to warrant him being placed in intensive care. He had just finished chemotherapy so his body was immunosuppressed and unable to fight on its own. I figured he probably was septic, meaning the infection was in his blood stream. This combination of immunosuppression and sepsis is often life threatening. I knew he was at the best place he could be, in a world class hospital. Yet, I felt so helpless. The hospital had recently started a program where friends and family members could send e-greetings to patients. I decided this was something I could do to show Ivan I cared. At that point I had never even talked to him on the phone. My e-mail said-

Hi Ivan, I was so bummed that you got sick again and ended up back in the hospital. I was so looking forward to meeting you yesterday. Hopefully this is just a bump in the road and you'll be out soon. If there is anything that I can do for you or your brother let me know and I will do my best to help. I'm looking forward to meeting you when you feel up to it. Cindy Locke

I had been told that Ivan had just received a laptop computer for his Make-A-Wish gift. I was hoping that he would be able to send me an e-mail back. I knew with his shyness, a phone call was probably out of the question.

I was antsy all week, wanting so badly to visit him at the hospital, but knowing I just needed to be patient. Later that week, I was happy to have the diversion of our local county fair. Each year the family would move our tent trailer to the back parking lot of the

Evergreen State Fair and live there on and off for five days. Jordan would enter his rabbit herd into the 4-H competition, and the girls would enter their flock of chickens. When the kids weren't busy with competitions or caring for their animals, we would wander the fairgrounds until we got tired and then go eat or rest in our tent trailer. Since we live only a half hour drive away, we would often go back and forth between the fair and home. Every night either Lenny or I would stay in the tent trailer with a various combination of the kids. It was a fun summer activity we had been doing for the past several years. Each day when I went home I'd check the answering machine and e-mail hoping to find a message from Ivan, none came.

The following Monday I received a call from the oncology social worker. I had met this social worker five years earlier when we did foster care for a baby with cancer and his teenage mother. She shared that now, one week after Ivan had been admitted to the hospital, he was doing much better, on a regular medical unit, and able to meet me. We made plans to meet the following day. The social worker decided she would be there to introduce us after reiterating that Ivan was very shy and quiet.

The following day, as I prepared to meet Ivan, I was very nervous. It had been almost a month since I had first heard about him. My mind had imagined, guessed, wondered, and worried every day about this boy. As I parked and found my way to a new medical floor, my anticipation grew. How would he receive me? What if he doesn't like me? I finally found his room and could see the social worker through the window. I entered cautiously. There he was, the boy that I had thought about so much and prayed for constantly since I had heard about him. He was sitting on his hospital bed, very pale, with no hair or eyebrows. He had a nasogastric tube coming from his nose and next to him sat a pink basin. I could only imagine that he was still nauseated from the chemo that he had recently finished and also the illness that he was still fighting. He looked so young. Though he was almost 16, I would have guessed he was maybe 13 or 14. Unlike his brother who showed traits of his Native American ancestry, Ivan looked like a very pale Caucasian boy.

After the introductions, the social worker and I chatted briefly and then she excused herself from the room. Ivan had only glanced up at me a couple times and kept his shoulders hunched. With his head down he looked primarily at the bed. I spoke to him and he would only nod or shrug his shoulders. He used no words and made no eye contact. I noticed the folder of pictures that I had sent sitting near his bed. Feeling awkward and not knowing what to say next, I grabbed the folder, sat down next to him, and started talking about our family. I described Lenny and the kids, their personalities, hobbies and interests. I described what our family liked to do together and how our house was laid out. I told him about his room, and how it was downstairs near Jordan and Josiah's room and that the girls were all together in the upstairs bedrooms. I talked about random family facts. Ivan said nothing; he would just glance at the pictures and continue to look at the bed. Shy and quiet was an understatement when it came to describing Ivan. I rambled on for the next half hour or so feeling somewhat ridiculous, wondering what Ivan was thinking about me. Was he thinking, "I wish this lady would just shut up and leave." I had no idea. He gave me no verbal or non-verbal cues.

Just before I started to leave I was telling Ivan about our friend's baby, Brent, and his battle with cancer. Ivan, out of the blue, said "Do you want to see my scar?" This was the first thing he had spontaneously said during the entire meeting.

"Sure," I said and he lifted his shirt to show me the six inch scar that ran down his spine. I ran my hand over his back and could feel the uneven spine where part of it had been removed to get to the tumor. I was amazed that he was willing to show this to me. I felt at that moment he had opened the door to his world, even if just a crack. At the same time I also felt so much sadness as I thought of him going through surgery alone. As I stood to leave, I felt compelled to hug him. Not knowing if this would freak him out, I decided to take a chance like I did with his brother a week before. To my surprise, when I hugged him he hugged me back. I had expected him to be a "limp fish" with his arms down to his side and me doing the hugging. As he returned my hug I wondered if maybe he wasn't as shut down emotionally as he appeared, maybe I could reach him.

I felt good when I left the hospital. I liked this kid even though he didn't talk to me. I saw him as a mystery and a challenge. Somehow, I'm going to get him to open up, show the real Ivan that I knew lay within. I wasn't sure how I was going to accomplish that feat. He didn't really talk to his caseworker whom he had known for two years, and from what I heard from the social worker, he didn't talk to the hospital staff that he had known for a year. I decided somehow I would find a way into this boy's closed up heart.

Two days later Jami, Ivan's caseworker, flew down from Alaska. She had come to be present when he went through his end of treatment scans that were scheduled for the following day. Ivan was finally discharged after ten days of IV antibiotics he had received for his infection. Jami drove Ivan to our house to meet the whole family. This was also her opportunity to meet us all in person. I could see the weakness Ivan was still battling as he got out of the car. He now wore a hat to cover his bald head, he still had the NG tube hanging from his nose.

Ivan and Jami both entered the house after introductions were made with the family in the driveway. I attempted to show Ivan around the house. I took him to his room, hoping to get some reaction. He stood in the doorway of his new room and gave a slight nod of his head. It was curious to me that he didn't even want to go in, look around, or sit on the bed. I was still trying to read his body language but it was nearly impossible. The only thing I could tell was that he needed to sit instead of continuing the tour to the upstairs.

He had used his wheelchair most of the time unless he was in his room at the Ronald McDonald House. I would later find out his room there was like any standard hotel room. The rooms were comprised of two queen size beds, a small bathroom, closet, TV on a stand, and a window seat with storage below and on the sides. The size of the room didn't lend itself to much walking. Ten steps to the bathroom from his bed, two steps to the T.V., and that was about it. Our house is about 3,500 square feet on two floors; a bit more walking would now be required.

After the partial tour we all went to the rec. room and Ivan sat stiffly on the couch. Lenny and the kids all looked at him and each other as Jami and I sat and talked. I tried to get Ivan involved with the conversation by asking him questions. He shrugged and nodded, but did not speak. He continued to keep his eyes down with only occasional glances around the room. He did smile a couple times, but never allowed his teeth to show. His shoulders remained hunched with his hands clasped in his lap. He looked so uncomfortable, I just wanted to nudge him and say "relax a little." The kids gradually slipped out of the room and Lenny stepped away to work on the computer as Jami and I continued to talked. I'm sure they also felt the awkwardness and were happy to get away to break the tension. Jami and I made plans for meeting up the following day as we accompanied Ivan to his end of treatment scans. Their total visit to our home was brief, only about a half an hour. As Ivan walked to the car, I patted him on the shoulder and told him that I'd see him tomorrow. He did not respond.

I was anxious to see Ivan as I drove myself to the hospital the next day. I was also curious to see how Ivan and Seneca interacted together since he was going to be with us for the entire day. Ivan's end of treatment scans consisted of an ultrasound, MRI, CT scan, and bone scan. When they were complete we would meet with his physician and other staff members to go over the results of the scans and his care needs.

Scan days are long and tiring as they last most of the day. Jami and I met up near the admission desk. Ivan and Seneca were running late. This gave Jami and I a chance to talk face-to-face without Ivan present. I asked her more questions about his family history and the reason for his placement in residential treatment. I still had very little information on Ivan's background. She gave somewhat vague answers as she fielded my questions. It appeared that she was attempting to protect confidentiality while at the same time giving me information that would be helpful to me in providing care for Ivan.

She explained that Ivan's mother had been out of the picture since he was nine. One day she was there the next day she was gone, with no good bye and no further contact. Her parental rights were not severed, but she was not a resource for Ivan and had no contact with him. Abuse and neglect were a part of Ivan and Seneca's life as they had grown up. His father had been the bread winner of the family, and at times was not very involved in rearing his two boys.

About two years after Ivan's mother left the family, a new step- mother entered the picture. Ivan, then age eleven, quickly spiraled downhill emotionally. Shortly after her arrival to the family Ivan was placed in a psychiatric facility. He was then transferred to residential treatment facilities first in Alaska then in Montana. Ivan had attempted suicide on at least two different occasions. He had been moved around to different institutions for a total of four years. Two months before his cancer diagnosis he was finally able to move out of the residential treatment facility. His father had refused his request to come home, so he was then placed in a group home back in Alaska. The month before Ivan was diagnosed with cancer, his father chose to relinquish his parental rights to Ivan.

As his life story was summarized, my heart broke. No child should have had to live through what Ivan had. Jami said that Ivan had done well in residential treatment and he was liked by the staff. Even though the staff felt Ivan would do better continuing to live in a group home rather than a foster family, Jami believed he would do well in a home environment. She was willing to try for a home placement. The only other option was to place him in a group home in Alaska and fly him back and forth to the hospital for his follow-up care. I was hoping that she was right, and that he would cope well in our family.

Seneca and Ivan finally arrived to where we

were waiting a short time later. Seneca was pushing Ivan's wheelchair. They had come across the street and up the hill from the Ronald McDonald house to the hospital. This was a trip that they surely had made hundreds of times before for appointments, school, therapy, and admission to the hospital. Seneca had a different appearance from our first meeting. He had buzzed his long hair off in an attempt to make Ivan happy during his last hospitalization. I'm not sure Ivan really cared if Seneca had long or short hair, but at least Ivan had company being bald.

The four of us headed off to get Ivan checked in for his scans. Seneca continued to push Ivan, with Jami and I feeling like unnecessary tag-a-longs. The two of them had done this before and knew exactly where to go and what to expect. Jami and I mainly followed and observed. Between scans we would sit in the waiting room until the staff was ready to put Ivan through the next test.

I watched Seneca and Ivan. There was not a lot of talk between them but they were always playfully jabbing, punching, or slapping each other. They seemed to communicate to each other with glances, head nods, and raised eye brows. It was a communication style that I had never seen before. I was completely fascinated watching their interactions. You could tell they were talking to each other without even saying a word. I was somewhat jealous seeing them communicate and not being a part of it. The bond the two of them had was obvious. Ivan was comfortable with his brother. I hoped that someday he would feel comfortable enough to communicate with me.

Later that afternoon we waited anxiously for the results of the scans. The team of medical personnel, who had worked to save Ivan's life, along with Ivan, Seneca, Jami and I crowded into a meeting room that was far too small for all of us to fit in comfortably. Ivan kept his head down and didn't speak during the meeting. He'd nod or shrug his shoulders when asked questions by the staff. If his cancer was still present it would have been a death sentence. With a big sigh of relief, we learned that his scans were clear. They could not see any cancer present in Ivan's body. He was done with his cancer treatment and ready for discharge. The only thing that would need to be followed was a blood clot that had not been fully resolved. He would need to continue on a twice a day injection of blood thinner. He would also need to be monitored for his weight since he'd had difficulties keeping weight on over the past several months. Follow up scans would need to be repeated every three months for the foreseeable future.

After the meeting, we made plans for Seneca and Ivan to come the following Monday, which was Labor Day, for a barbeque at our house. I really wanted Seneca to meet the family and see where his brother would be living. I hoped that he would feel comfortable enough to come and hang out with his brother at our house after Ivan moved in.

On Labor Day afternoon I picked up the two brothers. I wondered how the kids would react to Seneca. I had told them that he had multiple piercings, and tattoos, things they had not seen much of before. That day Seneca also wore jade jewelry that went through the septum of his nose. The jewelry looked like horns protruding from his nostrils. It was impressive to our family who had not been exposed to this form of body art. The kids were friendly but quite reserved around both Seneca and Ivan. There was tension in the air as we all tried to make small talk. Ivan sat stiffly on the couch, with Seneca next to him. The two of them would occasionally talk to each other, but still Ivan said nothing to the rest of the family. Seneca would talk to us, but the conversation didn't flow easily.

Lenny and Jordan were busy barbecuing the hamburgers and steaks. I had prepared the side dishes before going to pick up the brothers. When the meat was done I called everyone in to eat and Lenny prayed a blessing over the food. We set the food up buffet style around our big kitchen. I asked Seneca and Ivan to go first, since they were our guests. Seneca grabbed a plate and started filling it. Ivan just stood there. I encouraged him again. He stood there seemingly paralyzed. Awkwardness grew as the kids anxiously waited for their turn to go through the kitchen. Ivan remained unable to move or speak. Why was getting a plate and filling it with food so overwhelming to him? I grabbed a plate and started asking what he wanted, pointing to each choice of food, all the way around the kitchen. He was only able to nod a simple yes or no as I asked him about each dish. It seemed that this simple task of loading his plate had triggered a response similar to a panic attack. I hurt for Ivan. What had he experienced in his life to have caused such a reaction?

After the two of them had their meals, the rest of the family loaded our plates and joined them on the patio. The conversations remained stiff while we ate, with Seneca doing most of the talking and Ivan nodding or responding with one word answers. Shortly after the meal was over, and with the tension and awkwardness exhausting, I decided to take them back to the Ronald McDonald House. On the trip back I made a point of asking Ivan questions that were impossible to answer with just one word. "What's your favorite subject in school?" "What is it about that subject that you like?" He reluctantly answered my questions with as few words as possible or he just shrugged his shoulders. At least I got to hear him speak a couple phrases. That was an accomplishment. I felt we had made some progress, however small.

The following day I spoke with Jami, who by this time was back at her office in Alaska. We had not received the approval for Ivan to officially move to our house. I was unaware of the difficulties that we would face in getting approval for him to move into our home. In Ivan's situation there were two states with multiple layers of bureaucracy that had to work together to make the placement official. Surely by the end of the week all the red tape would be figured out. He no longer needed to be at the Ronald McDonald house since his cancer treatment was over. Other children and their families were in need of his room. On top of all this, the new school year had just begun. Ivan needed to get started so that he wouldn't feel like he was so far behind. Jami assured me that she would be making calls to try to get the approval finalized for his placement. Meanwhile, we were given the green light to bring Ivan home for visits as much as possible. The only stipulation was that he needed to be brought back to the Ronald McDonald House each night. Later that day I called and Ivan answered the phone. With the fewest possible words we were able to make plans for me to pick him up the following afternoon so he could eat dinner and hang out with the family.

As I drove to get Ivan I prayed fervently. I so badly wanted Ivan to feel accepted, comfortable, and loved by our family. I wanted him to be able to be who he was created to be. I arrived at the Ronald McDonald house and was buzzed in through the security door. I asked the staff at the front desk to let Ivan know I was there to get him. Within minutes he slowly walked down the hall into the large lobby where I was standing. I noticed that he no longer had the nasogastric tube. As he approached he made eye contact for a brief moment then put his head back down. I said hello and patted his back. "Ready to go?" Without an answer we headed for the car.

Later in the car I asked Ivan "What happened with your NG tube?"

"It fell out and I didn't feel like putting it back in." He replied. It was my guess that he had helped it "fall" out.

I wondered if the staff at the hospital knew that he no longer was being tube fed. His weight had been barely acceptable, even with the extra nutrition of the tube feeds. I decided not to ask more questions about the NG tube. We drove the rest of the way to the house with me talking and Ivan listening and nodding.

Ivan had been tied to the hospital and the Ronald McDonald house for the entire year. Seneca had bought himself a new car in Alaska just prior to being asked to come and care for Ivan in Seattle. He was never able to get the car shipped down, so the two of them had no vehicle. Their only means of transportation had been

the bus except for the few times when others had offered
to drive them to where they needed to go. Between
recovering from the paralysis and dealing with the
effects of the chemotherapy and radiation, Ivan was
usually too sick and weak to take the bus. Just the ability
to get away from the hospital and see a new place was a
treat for Ivan, even if it was uncomfortable to be with a
person he hardly knew.

We arrived at the house. The kids cautiously
said "Hi" as Ivan made his way to the couch in the rec.
room where he had sat the other day with his brother. He
looked pale and uncomfortable as he sat there staring
blankly at the TV that was off. "Do you want to watch
some TV?" He shook his head, no. It hurt to watch him
sitting there feeling emotionally and physically
uncomfortable.

"Do you have a bucket?" He asked.

"Are you feeling sick?" I questioned.

"Yes." He replied.

I quickly headed off to find a "puke bucket"
hoping I would return in time. I gave him the pink
hospital basin to keep nearby. Without asking I grabbed

his legs and swung them around until he was lying on the coach and put a pillow under his head. I removed his shoes and set them aside. He didn't resist any of my care and seemed to relax somewhat after he was lying down for a while. I tried to encourage him, "This is going to be your home. I want you to feel comfortable here. You can lie down on the couch, it's your couch now too."

How would I get him to feel like a member of the family and not a guest? For him to recover he would need to be able to relax in this house. He would need to be able to feel comfortable rummaging through the cupboards or the fridge, lying on the couch, and many other ordinary parts of living in a family. Ivan had been living in institutions for so many years, where he was undoubtedly told what to do and when to do it. I'm sure it would take time for him to feel comfortable and be able to move about freely like a family member.

The family tried to go about our regular evening routine of doing homework, eating dinner, and cleaning the kitchen. Ivan stayed on the couch looking, and most likely feeling, quite out of place. No words, no eye contact, and no smiles make for a difficult time getting to know another person.

Later that evening while driving Ivan back to the Ronald McDonald house, I was filling up the dead air with idle chit chat. Ivan sat quietly in the seat next to me. "Can you pull over please?" he said with urgency. I quickly pulled my green Subaru to the curb. He opened the door and threw his legs out of the car. He sat there with his elbows on his knees and began to retch and vomit. This had been his life for the past year. Feeling ill most of the time, afraid to go places, not knowing where and when you might need to vomit. I sat there not knowing what to do for him. I didn't want him to think I was babying him, but I didn't want to ignore him either. I reached over and gently rubbed his back as he continued to heave. He took off his knit hat that he used to hide his bald head as he broke out in a hard sweat. I had not seen his bald head since the first day I had met him. Waves of sorrow hit me as I imagined the emotional and physical suffering that he had endured over the past several years while mostly alone. It was clear to me that though he was nearly sixteen, he still needed a mom to comfort him.

Cindy Locke

CHAPTER 3

Over the next several weeks, as we waited for the two states to communicate with each other and untie the red tape, I continued to drive Ivan back and forth to our house. Seneca was working five evenings a week at a tattoo and piercing shop so I never saw him. I picked Ivan up right after Seneca left for work and would return Ivan before he got home. I continued to talk seemingly to myself as I drove with Ivan. Every night he was with us, he would have dinner. He was getting better about being able to load his own plate, but he still wasn't eating much food at all. Often I'd quiz him about what he had eaten since I'd last seen him. His response might be something like, "Top Ramen and a pickle." Since he no longer had his NG tube for added nutrients and calories, I was quite concerned about him losing drastic amounts of weight. I calculated the approximate calories a day he was taking in at around 500-1000. This was not nearly enough to keep weight on his thin frame. The following week he had a scheduled check up at the oncology clinic. I hoped that his nurse practitioner could give me ideas of how to help Ivan eat adequate amounts of food.

One evening after I drove Ivan back, I asked if he could show me his room. He hesitantly said ok. At that time I had only seen the lobby of the Ronald McDonald house and nothing else. I'd been impressed with the facility, it was beautiful like a five star hotel. We passed through the lobby, a family TV area, by a computer room, and finally up a ramp and down a hall to his room. As I entered, I was shocked by the amount of stuff they had packed in their room. The room was the size of a standard hotel room with two queen beds. About 90% of the floor was covered. Just a small path led to the beds and the bathroom. Ivan had lived in institutions for the past 4 years, and all his earthly possessions had followed him with each move.

I looked around the room at the mixture of their belongings. There was his wheelchair and ten cases of formula for NG feedings. Boxes of feeding bags sat next to a box of toys and books that looked like it belonged to an 8 or 9 year old. A bag of garbage sat next to several pairs of shoes. Medical supplies, his laptop computer, dirty clothes and half eaten food lay on his bed. The bed had multiple stains where formula had spilled and dried, it smelled horrible. This was definitely a bachelor's pad and it had been Ivan and Seneca's home for an entire year.

I noticed some photo albums lying on his bed side table and asked if I could see a picture of him before he got sick. We cleared a spot on the bed and sat together as he found some pictures of himself just prior to being diagnosed with cancer. What a handsome healthy teenager he had been. Light brown, collar length, wavy hair framed his handsome face. He had been full of color with freckles across his cheeks, whereas now he was ghostly pale. There was very little resemblance between what he looked like only one short year ago and now.

We continued through the photo albums with me making comments of how cute he was as a baby, toddler, or small child. He had such a sparkle in his eyes with real smiles when he was younger. There were pictures of him and Seneca playing on the beach and at a carnival. There were several pictures of him with his father and mother when he was about 7 years old. We looked through pictures of parents, grandparents, uncles, and cousins along with Ivan and Seneca at large family gatherings. Everyone was smiling and looking like the All-American middle class family at Thanksgiving or Christmas. The pictures were so confusing to me. With such a large extended family that appeared so loving in each photo, why were Ivan and Seneca all alone in this horrible situation, dealing with life and death by themselves? Ivan answered my basic questions with the fewest words possible,

"Who is this?" I'd ask.

"My Uncle." He answered.

"How old were you in this picture?"

"About eight." He replied.

He did not elaborate, but seemed to be happy to share that part of his life with me. I wondered what it felt like to looking back at pictures of happier times. For me, I hurt even worse for Ivan after seeing what he had lost: his handsome looks, his beautiful hair, his family, his support. I gave Ivan a big hug, encouraged him to keep eating, told him I'd be back the next day to get him, and left. I so badly wanted to just bring him home with me right them. Why does the foster care system have to be so ridiculously slow sometimes?

After three weeks of being ready for discharge, several calls to our state representative's office were needed to un-jam the paperwork processing. I was finally able to call Ivan at the Ronald McDonald house. "We got the ok. I will come and get you this evening after dinner."

"Ok." is all I got from Ivan.

"Can you call Seneca on his cell phone and let him know that you will be moving out tonight?" I requested.

"Ok." He answered.

I wasn't sure how Seneca was going to do with

his brother moving out. I couldn't tell if he was going to be relieved because the burden of Ivan's care would be off his shoulders and he could go back to being a free spirited twenty three year old, or if he felt he was losing his closest friend. Maybe a little bit of both. I also couldn't tell if Seneca was avoiding me or truly busy working and attempting to get settled in an apartment somewhere. The lines of communication were shut down as I had not seen him nor spoken to him since he came to our house for dinner three weeks earlier. Ivan had Seneca's cell phone number and I did not. All messages were passed to Seneca through Ivan.

I arrived that evening and began helping Ivan pack the piles of his belongings into boxes and black garbage bags. The Ronald McDonald house had the same kind of luggage carriers that you find in hotels. We piled it high several times over and filled our minivan. The exertion of doing this was exhausting for Ivan. I was still loading the van when he slipped around to the passenger seat. I noticed he was sweating and very pale.

"You feeling sick?" I asked.

"Yes." He managed to reply.

By that time, I had added a gallon size zip lock bag to my purse. I grabbed it and gave it to him as he sat there and heaved. I felt bad that I hadn't noticed his fatigue before he got to this point. I could tell that not only was getting sick unpleasant, Ivan was trying so hard to be just a typical teenager. He so badly wanted to leave the cancer, chemo, and hospital life behind. In his mind, he was done with anything that had to do with cancer or sickness. It was now time for Ivan to move on and have a regular life in a regular house with a regular family.

After the van was packed as full as we could get it and Ivan was feeling better, we made the trip home. I was so excited this day had finally come. I had known about Ivan for nearly two months by this time, and had met him about a month prior. Those two months were very long, but as I look back on the experience I'm glad the process went at a slower pace than we had expected. Ivan was able to gradually separate from Seneca and slowly get to know us. I think it was kinder to his psyche than just moving him in right after we met.

When we arrived, the whole family came out to help us move all the boxes and bags into Ivan's room. I knew unpacking would be too physically taxing for Ivan, so I joined him in his room to help. As I helped him go through the boxes and bags, I asked a lot of questions. You can find out a great deal about a person by their belongings. Seeing what someone likes, and what is meaningful to them gives a person insight into another person's soul. As I asked questions he began sharing some of the stories of his life; stories of his childhood. At first the stories were not too personal. He shared about books he liked to read as a child, games he liked to play. The evening wore on and we both became more and more tired of the unpacking process. In his things was a fiber optic Christmas tree he had received that prior Christmas. He began taking it apart. When he took the fiber optic part of it off, it shone psychedelic colors on the ceiling of his room. I turned the light off and we lay on his double bed exhausted, looking up and watching the colors flash around.

"My step mom used to make me sleep on the garage floor when she was mad at me." He said it with little emotion. "She wouldn't even let me come in to use the bathroom. Sometimes I'd go outside and pee on her car." He paused. "If she knew I liked any of my stuff she would donate it to charity to punish me. She gave away my 50 states quarter collection." Painful stories began to flow out of his mouth as we lay there in the dark staring at the ceiling. I felt so privileged that he would allow me to look into his heart and see the pain he had stored there.

The next day we returned to the Ronald McDonald House to get the rest of Ivan's belongings. The room was still half full. We dug through the piles and boxes trying to pick out Ivan's belongings and separated them from Seneca's. As I went to the far side of the room, which primarily housed Seneca's things, Ivan seemed more anxious. I wasn't quite sure what was going on until I lifted a blanket off a pile sitting on the window seat. Under the blanket was an aquarium with a little gecko in it. "You weren't supposed to see that. We aren't supposed to have pets in the house. Seneca got it for me, his name is Flaming Pizza."

I found out later that Seneca loved reptiles. Along with leaving his new car, Seneca had left a large assortment of snakes, lizards, gecko's, and other creatures behind in Alaska when he had to suddenly move down to take care of Ivan in Washington. His reptiles were his "babies." Seneca really had given up everything for his brother. I wasn't about to go tell the management that the brothers had been breaking the rules. Their secret was safe with me.

By the time Ivan moved in with us he felt a little more comfortable in moving around the house. He still needed reassurance that it was okay to eat whatever and whenever he wanted. I was very concerned about his weight and was happy to have him eating. Even with my reassurance he could not bring himself to open the cupboards, go in the pantry or open the refrigerator. So to encourage eating, I took a plastic bin with a large selection of non-perishable food and placed it in his room. Until he felt comfortable digging through our kitchen, he could have his own supply.

It was still awkward for him to be around the other kids. He rarely spoke to them and they gave him a lot of distance. But one evening, after he'd been with us for two weeks, as the sun was beginning to set; the kids were playing Frisbee outside in the yard. Ivan quietly moved outside to watch. He sat on a bench observing as the kids threw disks to one another. Sometimes the kids would throw the Frisbee to him and eventually he was standing and playing with them. I could hear laughter and the sound of cheerful kids coming from the back yard. Running was impossible for Ivan and bending was difficult. Yet as I peeked out the sliding glass door, I could see Ivan shuffling around despite his stiff and weak legs. He was playing and he was having fun! Later Sarah ran in exclaiming "Ivan took off his hat!" This was the first time he felt safe enough to show his bald head to the kids. An hour and a half later six exhausted kids poured inside from the darkness. Ivan looked genuinely happy for the first time since I had met him. "I'm going to sleep good tonight," he said spontaneously. My kids told me this was the first time they felt truly connected. The boundaries that divided them ceased to exist as they threw the Frisbee to each other thinking only of the game. Little by little change was happening.

Shortly after Ivan arrived we enrolled him in school. We met with the high school staff and agreed on a shortened school day as Ivan's endurance was still low. Ivan had an IEP (individual education plan) in place from when he lived at the residential treatment center in Montana. This was frustrating to Ivan since he didn't think he needed one. He hated people thinking he was developmentally delayed in any way. Along with the

IEP, Ivan had to ride the "little bus," in the mornings because of his late start at school. In Ivan's mind, only kids with cognitive deficits road "the little bus" so he was completely embarrassed. I tried in vain to convince him that a lot of different students rode "the little buses" but he would not buy into my explanations. I had heard that Ivan had an extremely high IQ, bordering on genius. I knew the IEP was not in place for cognitive deficits. It did however make getting services easier and rules were lifted to accommodate him. Ivan was also given a key to the school elevator. He was still too weak to climb more than a few stairs.

Ivan didn't want anyone to know that he had just been through cancer treatment. Only the staff that was involved directly with him was told about his condition and they tried to keep it quiet. The school had a no hat rule but allowed Ivan to wear hats to cover his bald head. Even though he didn't want the teachers or students to know about his cancer it was pretty apparent. When a student arrives who is bald and has no eyebrows it is pretty obvious he'd just undergone some extensive medical treatment. His appearance alone told his classmates that he had cancer.

Ivan's first day of school I drove him and dropped him off in front of the school. After a quick goodbye and a hug he shuffled away from the car towards the school. I was more nervous for him going to his first day at this new high school than I had been for any of my kids on their first day of kindergarten. Ivan was physically weak and extremely shy. I didn't know how he would do or how the other kids would treat him.

That afternoon he rode the bus home with Jordan. The bus let him off several blocks away from the house but fortunately there is a slight downward slope. I knew the approximate time they should be arriving so I pretended to be weeding the flower beds right then. Soon the two of them sauntered down the road. Ivan was doing ok until he hit our driveway which has an upward slope. His energy spent, he stopped several times before he was able to finish the walk up. I took his backpack and walked next to him as he slung his arm over my shoulder for the rest of the slow walk to the house. Though he appeared quite tired, he had finished the first day of school with no terrible stories to tell. I was proud of him and his accomplishment. I think it had felt good to Ivan to be out going to a regular high school. For several years he had been either going to school at the residential treatment facility or at the hospital school. I was still nervous over the next few days as Ivan would head off to school on "the little bus," but soon began to realize that he could hold his own at the high school. I would continue to meet him at the bottom of the driveway, but soon he was able to make it up the small incline just fine and no longer needed my help.

One evening as I looked through his clothes to see what other items he might need. I noticed a very ratty looking snowboard jacket. It was dirty and stained; the cuffs were nearly falling off, hanging by just a couple inches of material. He had a couple of other jackets; one was made for wearing in -20 degree Alaskan winters. The other ones were in new condition but not as stylish as the snowboarding jacket. I asked him which jacket he would wear to school when it got cold. He indicated the snowboard jacket. I pointed out to him how worn out and dirty it was. Why would he choose this jacket?

"I don't care, when it gets cold that's the one I will wear." He stated. I was mortified. I hate when foster kids are treated poorly and made to wear ugly, worn out, or ill-fitting clothes. I didn't want to be seen as one of "those" types of foster moms.

"Can I take you out and buy you a new jacket?" I asked.

"No, I like this one." Ivan replied.

"Ivan, I don't think a homeless person would wear this jacket, it is falling apart." I stated.

"I don't care, I like it." He assured me.

The horror I felt as I imagined Ivan wearing this dirty, tattered coat to school was overwhelming. I knew Ivan liked money and I was desperate.

"Ivan, I will buy this coat from you for $10."

Ivan replied "$30?"

Me "$20."

We settled, and Ivan agreed to sell me his dirty, tattered jacket for $20. We then took it to the fire pit and had a ceremonial burning until it was a pile of ash. As we sat in lawn chairs watching it burn, Ivan shared that he had been given this jacket by another young man that he had looked up to. The young man had been living at the group home that Ivan was in when he was diagnosed with cancer. It made more sense to me why it meant so much to him when I heard the story. The next weekend I took him out and bought him an almost identical jacket. This one was clean and new.

A couple of weeks into school Ivan was still mostly shy and quiet. He was starting to talk a little more around the house, but very little in public.

One day after school Ivan said "I need to make a Toga."

"What for?" I asked.

"I can get extra credit if I wear a toga to class on Friday because we are learning about Greek gods." He replied.

For a kid who will hardly talk to people or look them in the eye I thought it funny that he would actually want to wear a toga to school to get a few extra credit points. So, we made a toga out of an old white sheet. That Friday I drove Ivan to school in his Toga. I laughed as he shuffled away, his toga was wrapped a bit tight and he had very little room to move his legs. The toga, along with the blue knit hat on his bald head and his high top tennis shoes made for quite a silly sight walking across campus. When he came home that afternoon he said that he and one other student were the only ones to actually dress up. This should have been my first clue that the real Ivan was nothing like the closed up introverted young man that we had been used to seeing around the house.

Medically speaking, Ivan was much easier to take care of than little Brent was when he was released for the hospital. I gave him an injection of Lovenox, a type of blood thinner, in the morning and again in the evening. Ivan didn't seem to mind receiving the injections. He didn't even wince. He did, however, hate the bruises they left behind. Ivan only wanted them done on his upper arms and would not allow me to spread the injections around to his abdomen or thighs because he was self-conscious of these bruises. The only other thing that I had to monitor was his weight. I took Ivan every couple weeks to the Oncology Unit at Children's hospital for weight checks.

It is a whole different world in the Oncology waiting room. Little bald kids wander about, some of them lively and talkative; others curled up on their parent's laps looking miserable. Many of those kids had the dreaded NG tube coming from their noses, while others had the outline of their Hickman Catheter showing under their clothing. On one visit I noticed an older teenager stride in, car keys in hand. As he checked in at the desk, I thought he looked pretty old to be a patient here. I wasn't sure he even was a patient because he appeared strong and healthy with a full head of hair. I continued to glance at him as he sat down across the waiting room. Then it dawned on me that it was Travis, the teenager that had Ewing's Sarcoma, the one I saw on the TV news. I couldn't believe he could have a terminal illness. He looked too healthy. I didn't say anything to Ivan, though I wondered if he had heard of Travis or his story.

Often we would have to wait a half hour to an hour for Ivan's appointment time. We learned many ways of entertaining ourselves as we waited. Ivan would always wear his iPod to appointments and most every other place we went. Ivan loved all kinds of music: hip hop, rap, Reggae, 80's rock. These were styles of music

I had always avoided and encouraged my other kids not to listen to. I didn't appreciate the swearing, violence, and sexual content that came with most of those types of music. I had to make different rules for Ivan. I had not raised him, and shunning his music would have been putting a large wall up between us. His music was one of the most important things in his life. Instead, I decided that I needed to understand the music and what made it so appealing to Ivan. So while we'd sit and wait Ivan would give me one ear bud and he'd listen with the other. My mouth would drop, eyes wide open as I'd turn to look at Ivan. He'd crack a smile as "F bombs" were dropped or disgusting sexual innuendos were sung. I think Ivan usually protected me from the worst of the songs, but once in a while he did like to pick a song that he knew would get a big reaction from me. I had a friend when I was a young adult who said that I made Snow White look evil. I think that statement could still be said about me as a 40 something year old woman. Over time I began to understand how the lyrics of the songs related to his life. I no longer only heard the cussing; instead I could hear what made the songs powerful to Ivan.

The primary medical person we saw was a Nurse Practitioner named Sue. Sue was a petite nurse with a strong, matter of fact personality. She had been working with Ivan the entire year and knew him well. After Ivan's NG tube had come out, he was dropping weight and it was glaringly obvious at each weight check. It was hoped that once he got into a family situation with plenty of food choices and accessibility to food, his weight would begin to stabilize and perhaps increase. Ivan however, was not concerned about his weight at all and was happy to be dropping some pounds. He had not moved much in the past year and had lost most of his muscle tone. He now saw this flabbiness as chubbiness instead of just being soft from lack of exercise. Ivan commented that he felt he had man boobs, which were not acceptable. No matter how much Sue and I nagged him about eating and keeping his weight up, he was unfazed. He hated to even be at the hospital and he really hated us making a big deal about his weight.

Sue decided, at one of the visits, that it was time for Ivan to have the NG tube put back in. Easier said than done when you have a teenager who, though quiet and introverted, had an extremely strong will. After 20 minutes or so of cajoling Ivan to let her put the tube in Sue gave up and handed me the NG tube to try at home.

I hated placing NG tubes when I worked at the hospital but it was a skill I knew how to do. I was willing to try convincing Ivan at home. However, Ivan never let that tube near his nose at the hospital or at home. He was done with medical intervention and he was making it clear by refusing the tube. After that appointment he began refusing more interventions, even down to being weighed. We still continued to go to the hospital for labs but he refused to be weighed. He was eventually placed on an oral blood thinner instead of the Lovenox shots. Ivan was happy to be on the oral doses because he could avoid the twice daily shots that gave him the ugly bruises on his arms. This change made him willing to put up with the blood draws to check if his blood levels were correct. However, these levels were much more unstable and needed to be checked frequently. So we were often at the hospital a couple times a week for blood draws.

The trips soon became more of a time to say "Hi" to staff members and patients he knew rather than focusing on medical procedures. During that time Ivan, was finding his voice. For the year he was an inpatient and living at the Ronald McDonald house, he rarely talked to the staff, other patients, or their families. I think Seneca was the only one Ivan would carry on a conversation with that year. During one of the appointments with Nurse Practitioner Sue, Ivan chatted away about different things that were happening in his life. At the end on the appointment Sue said "You know Ivan, you said more to me in this one appointment than you have said to me in the entire year you were a patient here!" I knew Ivan was changing but hearing it from Sue made me realize that other people were seeing it as well. The real Ivan was beginning to show up. He was nothing like the quiet, withdrawn, sick boy that had moved into our house just a couple months before. He was funny and happy, and much to everyone's surprise, there seemed to be an extrovert in there trying to come out.

It began with our rides home from the hospital. Those rides, that had been so uncomfortable at first, became over the top crazy and silly. Ivan used that time to invent songs to sing to me as we drove home. He would roll down the window and yell "Hi" or "What's up?" to people waiting at a cross walk or bus stops. The change was so fast I had to work hard to keep up with it. I enjoyed every minute even though at times I was so embarrassed by his talking to the people on the street that I put the window locks on.

At home one day Ivan decided he wanted to do mime when he found some white face paint. He painted himself and three of the other kid's faces, and the four of them headed to the street in front of our house to put on a performance for the traffic that drove by. Still bald with just a bit of fuzz growing back on his head, and legs still stiff and somewhat shaky, he did a mime act in front of the house. As I cooked dinner, I could hear drivers beeping their horns in acknowledgement of this interesting entertainment. I stood there in the kitchen laughing and nearly crying as I realized the miracle that was happening. My love for Ivan was growing. I was amazed and in awe of that remarkable kid.

I noticed that as the days went by Ivan began to hold his body differently. Whereas before he used to look at the ground with his shoulders slumped forward, now he stood taller and looked outward instead of downward. He could now make and keep eye contact. Ivan was also much more verbal, especially around the house; but he still communicated primarily with body language, looks, and touch far more than most teenagers do. Since the first day I met Ivan I frequently gave him hugs and pats on the back as I did with all my other children. Ivan responded to this and soon was very expressive with me. He often cuddled up to me on the couch and would hold my hand or hang his arm around my shoulders while I was working in the kitchen. However, this overt affection was unusual because of his chronological age. I had observed during the past 20 years of foster parenting, that kids often became stuck emotionally at the age they were when the trauma occurred. I believe for Ivan, the peak of his trauma occurred when he was between the ages of 9 and 11 years old. His hunger for affection was more like that of a little boy.

One evening after Ivan had been sitting with me holding my hand on the couch watching a television show, I asked Lenny, "What do you think about how Ivan cuddles up to me and holds my hand?"

Lenny replied, "I think he just needs a Mommy."

Simple yet true, during that window of time, Ivan just needed a Mommy and I was blessed to be it. Yet it was awkward when relatives would come over and see Ivan literally hanging on me. My niece's husband, Phil, who was in his mid-twenties at the time, was confused and a bit shocked by this behavior. He stated that he wouldn't have ever been affectionate with his mom when he was that age. I tried to explain to him how kids get stuck at younger developmental stages because of trauma, abuse, and neglect, and they need to move through certain developmental milestones to heal and move on. I'm not sure Phil understood or accepted my explanation, he just thought it was strange. His opinion shook me, but deep down I knew that for this time, Ivan just needed time with a mom whom he could hang on and sit with in order to heal from his past.

Mid October Ivan had his 16th birthday. The Christmas Ivan spent at the Ronald McDonald House he had received a paintball gun. He had never been able to use it because he was too sick and there was nowhere to actually shoot. Once he moved to our house, he and Jordan used it in the yard, shooting cans on stumps, but after a while that wasn't very exciting. So, as part of his birthday party I invited Seneca to go with Ivan and Jordan to an indoor paintball court. It was full of bunkers, things to hide behind, and places to run around while shooting at each other. Ivan and Jordan were very excited. I got permission from Jami and his doctors before making the arrangements. His doctors were a little concerned because of the blood thinners that he was on, but consented as long as he wore thick clothing and had protective head gear.

We had only seen Seneca once since Ivan moved in with us. I was looking forward to the brothers getting together as much as Ivan was looking forward to seeing him. We had set up a time to drive south to Seattle to pick up Seneca before going back north to Everett to the paintball court. I wondered how Seneca was doing. I rarely had an opportunity to speak with him. We didn't know where Seneca lived after moving out of the Ronald McDonald house. He was a bit hesitant to give an address. I figured he would tell me when he was ready, I didn't want to be pushy. It wasn't my place to force him to tell me where he lived or how he was doing, although I did wonder and cared about him.

Ivan was contacted several times by the Ronald McDonald House staff, during the first couple months he lived with us. Seneca's belongings were still in the room and they didn't know what to do with them. We would then call Seneca and he would say he would go get them. I offered to help with the van and transporting his things for him, but he told me he would take care of it. After multiple calls, Ivan and I ended up picking up his belongings and bringing them back to our house. I didn't know what to think about Seneca or his circumstances.

On the day of the paintball match, we were excited and looking forward to the day as we traveled to pick him up. What better way to celebrate Ivan's 16th birthday than to get together with his brother and do something he had been looking forward to doing for many months? We were supposed to meet in front of the tattoo shop where Seneca worked. We arrived at the designated time and waited. After a few minutes Ivan tried calling Seneca's cell phone. He didn't answer. A few minutes later Ivan tried again and Seneca answered saying he was too tired to go. Ivan passed on the message. I was furious. We had gone an hour out of our way to get him, plus he was disappointing his brother. I could not understand why Seneca would do such a thing. If only I knew then what was going on in Seneca's life. With my lack of understanding, the combination of anger and sadness boiled inside me. Ivan, Jordan, and I drove the hour ride in silence. The excitement had disappeared.

We arrived at the paintball court; rented a second gun and the boys went to a back room to start getting ready. There were several other men and boys in the back doing the same. Ivan was still almost bald. He had just a smidgen of peach fuzz on his head. I wondered how he would deal with being around people he didn't know if he had to take his hat off to get the face shield on. Jordan and Ivan were preparing to go on the court but were having a difficult time with the equipment. The men saw them struggling and stepped in to help. Ivan seemed awkward but was able to speak when needed. I moved to the viewing area to wait, not wanting to embarrass them by having their mom hanging around.

Their turn came and everyone headed out to the court. The players would divide into teams and each team went to different ends of the court. An alarm sounded and all of them would run for protection. Jordan sprinted and quickly took cover. Ivan, still stiff and weak walked as fast as he could to get behind something. He was shot instantly. It broke my heart. I watched several rounds as he would try to play the game, and each time he was the first one shot. The combination of Seneca not coming, and having to watch Ivan waddle around getting shot time after time with no way to hide, was too painful for me. I drove off in my car sobbing. The perfect birthday gift was disintegrating into a day of sadness.

When I returned later to pick them up, both boys seemed happy. Ivan was discussing different guns with the other guys, he didn't seem discouraged or upset. I didn't let on how distraught I had been over the day's events.

That evening we had a small family birthday party for him with our friends, John, Susan and their kids. You put a family of 8 together with a family of 6 and you have an instant party. Ivan was still quite shy with "outsiders", but Susan knew how to connect with him. She had lived in Alaska as a child and had traveled there as an adult. She could talk to him about places that were familiar to him. Being half Alaskan native herself, she could also imitate some of the ways the older Native Alaskan women would speak which made Ivan chuckle. They connected culturally in a way I couldn't. It was fun to watch the two of them interact and be silly. It reminded me to not take for granted the relationships we form with others. At this point in Ivan's life, he had lost all of his childhood relationships. To watch new friendships forming was precious; and yet I was still sad, confused, and upset that Seneca hadn't been a part of Ivan's special day.

CHAPTER 4

As autumn rolled on, I began doing my Christmas shopping. I always tried to be done with my Christmas shopping by Thanksgiving. I didn't like to have to fight the crowds; rushing around with hordes of people took the joy out of the season for me. Ivan still loved to go places with me. Even going to Wal-Mart was exciting. His answer was almost always, "yes" if I asked him if he wanted to come along.

One evening after dinner, Ivan and I went to do some Christmas shopping at Wal-Mart for the other kids. As we wandered around the toy department looking for a gift for Josiah, Ivan kept hanging his arm around my shoulder. This was common around the house, but now we were in public. Here was a 16 year old boy who was taller than me, hanging on me like a little child. I felt awkward but I didn't say anything at first. The longer he hung on me the more uncomfortable I became. I tried to nonchalantly get out from under his arm to no avail. I finally had to say, "Ivan, this looks weird, let go of me." He didn't care one bit what anyone was thinking and kept his arm on my shoulder. I kept trying to peel him off, but the more I tried the more he tried to stay right where he was. By now he was trying his best to embarrass me I am sure. I was laughing and trying to run away from him. He was trying to grab me so that he could walk with his arm around me. By this time the other customers, and those monitoring the hidden cameras in the store were probably wondering what was going on between the middle age woman and that teenage boy.

Ivan was silly and goofy and he found another thing that he could use to embarrass me. PDA at Wal-Mart was even better than yelling "What's up?" out of the car window. I was finally able to make it to the electronics department, which created a big enough distraction for Ivan to quit playing the "Let's embarrass Cindy game." What a funny guy, it was getting to the point I could never guess what random silly trick he was going to play on me next.

As we left Wal-Mart that evening we pulled to a stop near the main road. A man who I had seen quite often pan handling on the corner was there. I usually avoided eye contact with him and felt awkward as I waited for the light to change to green. I had never stopped to talk to him or given him money. As we waited for the light to turn green, Ivan rolled down the window of the car, grabbed a handful of coins and bills out of his pocket and handed it to the man. I didn't know what to say. Who was this kid, who had very little money but was willing to give it to a stranger? Who was this boy who had been institutionalized with a list of scary psychological diagnoses, yet was so willing to love me and the Wal-Mart panhandler? Who was Ivan?

In November, I got an e-mail from Jami saying Ivan's former therapist from the residential treatment facility was going to be in town and wanted to come over to the house and visit Ivan. I was happy and excited to have her come and see him and how well he was doing.

During the week prior to her coming it was also an opportunity for Ivan to tell me more about his time living in Montana. We looked through some of the pictures he had from his time there. We also looked online at the residential treatment facilities website and on Google earth. It hadn't been a horrible experience for him so he didn't mind revisiting it at all. He loved the horses and animals that were used for therapy. He loved swimming in the pool and helping to teach other kids to swim. He also talked about their de-escalation rooms and how the staff managed his, and some of the other kids' behaviors.

When the therapist came, Ivan retreated back to the quiet boy who didn't talk much. Even with him not acting his new normal "goofy" self we'd observed, she was still impressed with the changes that she saw. The therapist had found some of Ivan's journals that had been left at the center, and brought them to him. After their brief visit she left. I really wanted to understand Ivan more and read what he had written while in treatment. Initially he refused my request. He knew how much I wanted to read them, so remembering the coat he said, "I will let you have them for a price." I had created a monster by buying that old coat. After negotiating, I finally bought the stack of journals for $15. Sadly, most of the journals were nearly empty. However, I did find one entry that was touching. Three years earlier, when he was 13 years, old he must have been asked to describe what his dream Christmas would be like, he'd written....

December 17 - My Christmas future will be fun with family having lots of food, lots of presents and no arguing. It would be so fun. It wouldn't be a treatment Christmas. It would be a big family Christmas. I hope that happens someday. It would be really fun.

I couldn't imagine the loneliness he must have felt, forced to spend his Christmases without family and apart from everyone he knew. In some ways, I think the pain of isolation was even worse than the physical pain he felt from the cancer. When he and his brother were reunified, the loneliness he faced every day in treatment was gone. Despite being ill, Ivan was more at peace.

While in treatment multiple psychological diagnoses where placed on him. Conduct Disorder, Reactive Attachment Disorder, Mood Disorder, and

Post-Traumatic Stress Disorder were a few. He had been diagnosed with all these serious disorders, yet I hadn't witnessed any behavior issues. I had been around plenty of kids with these same diagnoses. At first he was overly shy and shut down, but that wasn't even present now. I asked Ivan if he felt like he changed much inside since he was in Montana. He said he felt like the same kid, but that they perceived him differently. It was hard to figure out if he had really changed and the treatment had worked, or if he was just in a different environment that allowed him to let go of some of the behaviors that he had needed to survive his earlier life. All I knew was that unless we were still in the "honeymoon phase", and he would be radically changing in the near future, he was one of the most funny, loveable, entertaining teenage boys that I had ever met. I was excited he was with us to have his first "big family Christmas" like the one he wrote about in his journals.

As Thanksgiving approached I encouraged Ivan to invite Seneca to come and celebrate with us. I had not had any contact with him since before Ivan's birthday. Ivan finally reached him and asked him to come. I was able to speak to Seneca directly when Ivan passed me the phone. We made plans for where and when to pick up Seneca. I was hopeful that this time Seneca would show up, and not cancel. Ivan was looking forward to seeing his brother.

When the day came, Ivan and I went to pick up Seneca in the University District of Seattle. He met us on a street corner so we didn't know which apartment he lived in. I wasn't exactly sure what was going on, perhaps he just didn't want us to know his address. If he didn't want us to know where he lived, that was his choice.

The bond the brothers shared was so evident. They went back to their way of non-verbal communication; poking at each other, eye brow raising, and head nods. At the house Seneca and Ivan hung out together playing the Wii or went into Ivan's room. Seneca went through some of the boxes we had picked up from the Ronald McDonald house and picked out a few items to take back with him.

When all the guests began arriving for dinner I could sense Seneca's discomfort. It was the first time he had met our relatives, and with his quiet and introverted personality type, I knew it would be uncomfortable for him. He seemed more comfortable playing with the kids of our family than interacting with the adults. The kids had no problem with this, they loved him and were drawn to him. He had no qualms about getting on their level and engaging with them. It was cute to see such a big, tough looking man playing with the kids and hearing their squeals of delight as he chased or hid from them.

The evening seemed to go well for Seneca and Ivan. I was optimistic that Seneca would start coming to the house more often. I hoped he would start feeling more comfortable with us. Just like Ivan had needed time to adjust and come to know this was his home; I wanted Seneca to have that level of comfort here too. But it was hard to get to that point if he didn't come to visit. Seneca was mysterious to me. I knew he had a huge heart for his brother, little kids were drawn to him, and he was soft spoken and gentle natured. Yet he was still so closed up and hard to get to know. I wanted to understand who he was. I wished that he would just give me a chance.

In December, Jami contacted Ivan and me to let us know that his uncle on his father's side was going to be getting married in February. The family had requested for Ivan to travel to California to be part of the wedding. Jami wanted Ivan to have either Seneca or myself travel with him. She made this request partly because Ivan was a minor, and partly because she wasn't sure who would be at the wedding, or if certain interactions might be potentially upsetting to Ivan. Since Ivan's father had relinquished parental rights, Jami had no obligation to help Ivan attend. However, Ivan was excited about the possibility of going and was hoping to go with Seneca. When he was finally able to reach his big brother, Seneca told Ivan that he would not be able to take the time off of work to make the wedding.

I could tell Ivan was disappointed. He contacted Jami in hopes that he would be able attend the wedding without me. He said he felt like he was taking his babysitter along if I came. Ivan felt he could handle the trip on his own. Jami was not at all convinced that this was a good idea. It had been many years since he had seen most of his relatives and a lot had occurred during that time. I was happy to go with him but unsure what his family would be like, or if I would be well received. The pictures in Ivan's photo album made me think they were your typical middle class family. I was interested in meeting them. Maybe I could put the pieces together better in my mind of what happened to Ivan. Even though Ivan was resistant to my accompanying him, he knew that Jami would not allow him to go otherwise. Once we determined I would accompany Ivan to California, Jami began working out all the logistics of the trip and getting the court's permission for him to fly out of state.

As we drew closer to Christmas it was a magical time. It had been a very stormy fall season. One storm had winds reach over 50 mph which made for extensive power outages. I loved storms and so did Ivan. I liked to sit and watch them with a cup of coffee or hot chocolate. Ivan, however, wanted to be out in them. At first when the winds were 25mph or so I wasn't as concerned about him. I knew the back yard didn't have trees close enough to potentially drop branches on him. Later in the evening, as the winds really picked up, Ivan took off into the back yard with a blanket to try to catch some wind. Ivan had a zest for life that was contagious and endearing. However, at that point I had to put a stop to his fun. All sorts of things were flying around, and it wasn't only branches I was concerned with but entire trees falling over. I was the party pooper and made him come back inside. His attempt at flying in the wind made me chuckle. After being a rehab nurse for 7 years, I had seen too many kids with head injuries and spinal cord injuries. Ivan just beat cancer and I didn't want a new injury for him to have to deal with due to him being out in this storm.

With that mighty wind storm and some early snow storms, schools had been kept closed most of the days since Thanksgiving. Ivan had been missing Alaska and all the snow up there. We quickly found out that he was a big playful kid anytime it would snow here. When Ivan awoke to the first snow of the season he took off running in the back yard in his basketball shorts, what he called his "wife beater" tank top and no shoes. Most kids like snow, but his love for it was even more intense than most. All six of our kids spent hours outside over those several weeks enjoying every bit of time they could be out in the snow. I was so thankful that particular winter ended up being an exceptionally snowy one. I loved being "stuck" at home with my kids, not able to leave, with none of them being able to attend school. Our days centered on hot chocolate, snowmen, sledding, and getting ready for Christmas.

The Christmas before, Ivan had spent it with

Seneca at the Ronald McDonald house. This was his first Christmas in a house with a family since he was 11 years old and I wanted to make it a special one. Our family continued with our pre-Christmas traditions. I decorated the house with our Christmas village and other Christmas decorations. The family went to our favorite tree farm to pick a Christmas tree, cut it down, and then ride the flatbed trailer with our tree to the top of the hill. There we drank hot chocolate and ate candy canes at the farm before returning home to set up the tree.

In order for this Christmas to be the best one for Ivan, I knew Seneca would need to be a part of it. I was sure, since he had come for Thanksgiving, and seemed to have a good time, he would come for Christmas. I encouraged Ivan to invite Seneca. Ivan could never reach him by phone, so Christmas went on without his big brother. Was he mad at us, uncomfortable at our house, or did he have other things going on in his life that were preventing him from being here? I wasn't sure. It was the big family Christmas that Ivan had written and dreamed about, minus Seneca.

CHAPTER 5

Jami had made arrangements to come down from Alaska to check on Ivan. She hadn't seen him since his end of treatment scans in the first part of September. It was worked out with Washington State to send a social worker out every month to check on Ivan, but we had not seen anyone so far. I had stayed in close contact with Jami mainly by e-mail, with occasional phone calls, so she had stayed caught up on his progress. I was in no great hurry to have a Washington State social worker come check up on Ivan. Ivan was still quite private. I'm sure he would have been irritated to have another social worker meddling in his business. He was trying to just be a typical teenager, not a foster child that needed to be checked on.

Jami arrived on a snowy day in January. School had been cancelled for the day because of the hazardous road conditions. The kids had spent the day sledding, building snow forts, and doing various other snow activities. The mood of the house was happy and playful. Jami had planned to take Ivan out with her that evening, but the roads were too treacherous. She had taken a rental car with four wheel drive from the airport, but even then had difficulty making it to our house on the hilly roads. Instead of attempting the roads again, she hung out with us drinking hot chocolate and eating special cookies that she had brought. The kids affectionately named her cookies moose poop because of their appearance.

Ivan's now funny, lively personality retreated to his more quiet and subdued personality with Jami in the house. He was more animated than when she was here in September, but not like he usually acted around the house. I badly wanted her to see the over the top, funny, happy kid that we had come to know and love. She had invested over two years of her life trying to do the best for Ivan. She even rode with him in the plane when he was airlifted down from the hospital in Alaska to Seattle Children's Hospital. She then spent the first couple of days with him until Seneca could make it down. From my perspective, Jami was much more attached to him than most caseworkers were to the kids in their caseload. Jami would ask Ivan questions about school or what he wanted to do in the summer and Ivan would give her the shoulder shrug. She asked about his desire to learn how to drive, another shrug. Do you want to get a part time job this summer? Shrug. The communication was impossible and frustrating to watch. At this point Ivan rarely communicated like this unless non-family members were present.

Jami would be flying back to Alaska the following evening. We needed to use this time to plan for things. Jami and I talked while Ivan listened quietly. "It is very difficult, if not impossible, for a teenager in care to get a driver's license. This is all due to liability. The only way that it usually can be done is if the teenager is adopted, or the foster parents have legal guardianship". Ivan, now being sixteen, had brought up learning to drive several times over the past couple months. It wasn't a burning desire of his, but it was something he was thinking about. Jordan had received his driver's license just prior to Ivan joining our family. Ivan could see the freedom driving brought.

There is such a lack of freedom for foster kids. They need permission from their caseworker to jump on the trampoline, permission to go paintballing, permission to go on school field trips, ride horses, go camping, leave the state, etc. etc. The older foster kids often feel like their lives are being controlled by a caseworker who they hardly know. Jami stayed for dinner that night and then returned to her hotel. The next day we had planned to meet with school personnel to talk about Ivan's classes for the up-coming semester.

After I got the other kids to bed I wandered into Ivan's room. He was attempting to take apart an old remote control car. I was anxious to speak with him about details that were still left to discuss with Jami before she went back to Alaska. With pen and paper in hand I started asking Ivan what was important to him.

"I want a copy of my birth certificate." I wrote that down. "I want a State of Alaska ID card so that I can buy things without paying tax." I wrote that down. We continued to talk about what he wanted, plans he would like to make, and things he wanted to do that we might need to obtain Jami's permission.

I was sitting at the head of his bed with one leg hanging down, the other bent up and on the bed. Ivan had been fiddling with the little motor as we talked. His answers to my questions had been coming less often. Then he sat down on the bed just in front of me, his body turned facing the foot of the bed.

"This is your life Ivan; you need to ask for what you want." With pen and paper still in hand waiting for Ivan to talk, I glanced up. Ivan's shoulders were jerking up and down. I couldn't tell if he was laughing or crying because there was no sound. I leaned forward to see his face. I got a glimpse of his face before he turned it. He had tears streaming down. I was a little confused since our conversation had been so factual and non-emotional. I couldn't figure out what had triggered this reaction. I laid the pen and paper aside and I began stroking his back. With that touch Ivan laid back against me and I wrapped my arms around him. His arms clung to my arms as his shoulder's continued to shake and jerk as he let out silent sobs. I tried to adjust how I was sitting and he clung even tighter, his whole body shuddering. Tears dripped off his face on to my arms.

"What's the matter?" I asked quietly, stroking his face. No answer. "Do you want to tell me what's bothering you?" His body continued to shake, tears streaming down his face. I could see that his grief was far too deep to put into words, so I just sat there holding him, wiping tears, feeling the silent sobs shake his body.

It was around 10pm when I went to speak with Ivan. An hour later I still sat in the same position holding him. One leg was completely numb and my back ached, but I didn't want to let go of him. He still clung tightly to my arms. His body had stopped shaking and he was letting out long sighs. I was concerned Lenny would come looking for me since I'd been gone awhile, and now it was the time we usually went to bed. I didn't want Ivan embarrassed to be seen by Lenny in this emotional state.

"Ivan, I'm going to go out for a while. When I come back I want you to try and tell me what you were feeling and thinking."

I unfolded myself and went to find Lenny. I told

him briefly what had happened and that I probably wouldn't be coming to bed for a while, I wanted to give Ivan time to process what just happened and try to verbalize what he was feeling.

I had given Ivan about ten minutes alone before returning to his room. He was sitting on the edge of his bed, puffy red eyes looking at the floor, shoulders hunched, hands clasped in his lap. I sat next to him on the bed, my hand rubbing his back. Just as earlier the tears had flooded down his face, now words to his feelings were tumbling out. Random thoughts and feelings just poured out of him. It was like a dam of pain, frustration, and anger that he had been stuffing down for many years finally broke loose and everything just came pouring out. Unlike our normal dialog where I ask a lot of questions to prompt him along, tonight everything just came out. Everything from personal family issues he had experienced, feeling like he was forced to go through chemotherapy, being pitied by his teachers because of his cancer, to not feeling like anyone trusted him since he was a little boy; it all came out like an emotional explosion. After an hour of heart wrenching sobs followed by an hour of gut wrenching communication, both of us were exhausted. Through the whole ordeal Ivan had not made eye contact with me once. As I got up to leave I pulled him up from his seated position on the bed and made him look me in the eye. I wrapped my arms around him and held him. He hugged me back with a weary hug.

As I crawled into bed next to a half sleeping Lenny, I couldn't quite believe what had just happened. The emotional breakthrough for Ivan that I had been hoping for had finally happened and in such a big way. Everything he had said raced around in my mind. My heart was so full of love for him. He was no longer my foster child, he was my son.

The next day the snow had melted off the roads just enough that schools decided to open. Jami arrived mid-morning to accompany Ivan and me to the meeting at school. Two months earlier Ivan was embarrassing me with his overzealous affection in public, but now he was over that stage and was acting like a normal teenager. He didn't want me or Jami walking anywhere near to him at school. We gave him a couple minutes head start and told him we'd meet him in the counseling center.

I tried to explain to Jami what had happened the

night before. It was almost too big for words. He had a breakthrough and I loved this kid. The original plan for Ivan to go and live with Seneca after six months living with our family was fading away. Communication with Seneca was difficult for both Jami and me. We weren't sure what his plans were or even where he was living. Ivan would talk with him once in a while on his cell phone, but Seneca had refused to come over to visit or even meet us at clinic appointments. I was confused and not sure what was going on with Seneca. I had made a promise to not keep the brothers apart. I wanted Seneca to be a part of Ivan's life, but I couldn't make Seneca stay in Ivan's life. At this point it looked like Seneca had disappeared off the radar screen. It wasn't until many months later that I found out what Seneca was going through after Ivan moved in with our family.

That afternoon, Jami, Ivan and I started the conversation about making his stay with our family permanent. The options were guardianship or adoption. Guardianship would allow us to sign consent forms and have less interaction with state caseworkers. Ivan would have more freedom because we would be able to call the shots. Adoption would mean he would officially be our son and we would be his parents. The thought was both exciting and scary to me.

Adopting a teenager was somewhat of a foreign concept. We had adopted Emily at 3 years old and Josiah at 4 years old. Lenny and I were comfortable with adoption but contemplating the financial responsibility of parenting a child who has cancer is daunting. Even though his cancer was not present at this point, we knew that the potential for its return was high. Even if the cancer never returned, the cost of the follow up scans that are necessary every three months is huge. The thought of affording the expense of his adoption and his medical bills was frightening. Ivan was now 16 and we knew there was adoption support available until he turned 18 to help pay the medical bills, but after that there were a lot of unknowns. I shared none of my fears with Ivan. He took in the information and told Jami and I that he would think on it. For him I'm sure he was weighing the emotional expense. Choosing to be adopted by our family was saying good bye to his dream to live with Seneca. If Seneca was able to get an apartment, the option for Ivan to live with him would no longer be available until he became an adult.

Over the next couple weeks Lenny and I began

to process the information for ourselves. We looked closely at the pros and cons of adoption, guardianship, and continuing to do long term foster care. For me it boiled down to a mother's heart, I loved Ivan like I had birthed and raised him. I would do whatever it took to prove my love for him. I would throw reason and financial safety out the window because he meant that much to me. Lenny had not formed as intense of a relationship with Ivan. He truly cared for him, but Ivan had not been emotionally vulnerable with Lenny like he had with me. Nevertheless, Lenny backed me. If Ivan chose adoption, then we would do it.

A month or so after Jami left she called to see if a decision had been made. I had not pushed the idea on Ivan, but rather let him have time to process all the thoughts and feelings he had about his options. I had been reading online stories of teenagers being adopted. Most of these pieces were "feel good" stories of teenagers and parents talking about how great the adoption had been for both parties. I printed out some of the articles and gave them to Ivan. With not much expression or conversation, he read them.

After Jami had called to inquire about our

decision, Lenny, Ivan, and I sat and processed the whole decision together. Freedom from being a "foster kid" and being managed by the state was quite appealing to him. Being able to get his driver's license, go places without the state authorizing it, etc. was also a big draw for him. Ivan's biggest concerns were that he didn't want his new birth certificate to say he was born in Washington, and he wanted to keep his last name. He expressed that he wanted to be our son forever and wanted our relatives to be his relatives. He also liked that he would get our inheritance, which made me chuckle. He wanted a family that wanted him and believed in him. By this time all the kids in the family adored Ivan. He knew he was loved and he was wanted. So with very little fanfare, Ivan said yes he wanted to be adopted. We all committed to take the plunge. Regardless of our fears, we all decided it was meant to be.

I called Jami back and told her that everyone had decided on adoption. She asked me to have Ivan call her separately to express his desire to be adopted. Ivan, still not great on the phone, or great with words, reluctantly called Jami. As Jami spoke to Ivan, Ivan answered her questions with as few of words as possible. "Yes, Uh huh" went the conversation. He told her "Yes" to her question of whether or not he wanted to be adopted. I knew he meant it, but the enthusiasm did not translate well over the phone.

With the go ahead from our family and Ivan, Jami began the process of making it possible for us to include Ivan in our family. The adoption process usually takes months. The first step was updating our home study, which in itself could take several months. There was the additional issue of Ivan being Native Alaskan. Permission had to be obtained from his tribe. We had never adopted a child who was Native American, but I had heard that getting approval could be very difficult and might take a long time.

As part of the adoption, Jamie asked me to take Ivan back to have a psychological evaluation. Less than 2 years ago Ivan had been institutionalized for behavioral and psychological problems. Prior to the adoption they had to prove he was psychologically ready to become part of a family. Ivan hated going to see counselors and psychologists. He had attended evaluations and counseling since he was a small boy and disliked having to go again. I had no concerns over Ivan's behavior, or any concerns with him being depressed or suicidal. To me, he was perfect.

The only reason I looked forward to having the psychological evaluation was to have some of the labels that they had placed on him removed. One of his diagnoses was Reactive Attachment Disorder. I was very familiar with this diagnosis. We'd had a foster daughter for many years who was diagnosed with this same disorder. We had also worked as a "practice family" as children went through two weeks of intense therapy sessions with counselors who specialized in Reactive Attachment Disorder Therapy. Some of the symptoms that children with Attachment Disorder have are: they can be very charming to strangers, not affectionate on parents' terms, they can be cruel to animals, they frequently try to triangulate adults, and they lack conscience development just to name a few. Kids with severe Reactive Attachment Disorder have been known to kill pets, and even people with no feelings of remorse.

After living with Ivan for 6 months, I was absolutely sure this diagnosis was wrong. I felt such a deep connection to Ivan. I knew he had a conscience, he was affectionate and not manipulative in any way, and he was kind and gentle to our dog and the younger kids in the family. I was determined to have the psychologist remove that label from him.

Prior to the appointment I wrote a long letter to the psychologist he was scheduled to see. I went into great detail about Ivan's behavior in our family. I was concerned that Ivan would show up at the appointment and once again shut down. If he refused to speak except in one word answers, the psychologist might assume he was still depressed, avoidant, or uncooperative. As far as I could tell, Ivan was just shy around people he didn't know well, and he had no desire to share his inner world with yet another psychologist.

On the day of the appointment I spoke briefly with the psychologist before he met with Ivan privately. He thanked me for sending the letter in advance. I explained that Ivan was reluctant about meeting with him. I also mentioned my hopes Ivan would share some of his feelings and the psychologist would get a true picture of this wonderful young man.

I returned to the waiting room and began reading some random magazines. While waiting, the oncology social worker who had introduced Ivan to me several months earlier walked into the waiting room. I said "Hi" and struck up a conversation with her, telling her how well Ivan had been doing both medically and emotionally. I told her that our family had fallen in love with him and were beginning the adoption process. Her face looked confused and stunned, not happy and excited as I had imagined. There was a long quiet pause before she said "You do realize that his chance of survival is very low?" It was my turn to look confused and stunned. "Yes, I know the odds are bad. But we love him and want him to be part of our family. We want to walk through whatever happens as a family, not just his foster family." She said something kind and headed back to work. That was a reality check that I wasn't expecting. He was my boy. Having a poor prognosis didn't change anything about how much I loved him. Cancer or no cancer I wanted him as my son.

Ivan and I were required to return to see the psychologist two more times, which was very frustrating for Ivan. The psychologist acknowledged that Ivan seemed to be doing well at this point. He did warn me that the best indicator of future behavior is past behavior. With Ivan's extensive psychological history he could not assure me that he would continue to do well behaviorally. I listened to his opinion, but it did not change the way I saw him. Ivan was still perfect in my eyes.

All the plans had been made for Ivan and me to fly to California and attend Ivan's uncles wedding. I was excited and a bit nervous to meet all of his relatives. His parents would not be there, but all of his uncles, grandparents, cousins, and other distant relatives would be attending. Jamie had filled everyone in on our plans to adopt Ivan. I had spoken to Ivan's grandmother on the phone prior to traveling and she seemed accepting of me. I hoped that the rest of the family would be willing to accept me also. Along with airplane tickets, the state of Alaska provided us with a rental car and a hotel room. When we arrived we picked out the sportiest of all the cars available. Even though it was February, the weather was very warm as we drove around with our windows down. Ivan picked a rap station and cranked the volume up as we went looking for our hotel. Funny kid, didn't he know it wasn't cool to be doing that with his "mom" in the car? We checked into our hotel room and unloaded our luggage.

Shortly after we arrived, we were to meet at the

church for the wedding rehearsal. We parked on the street near the church watching for anyone who might be a relative. I was nervous and I could sense Ivan was also. He hadn't seen most of these relatives for many years. We waited until he saw a man walking outside of the church. Ivan said, "I think that's my uncle." He got out of the car and stood. His uncle came walking towards us. He asked, "Is that you Ivan?" then he hugged him. I introduced myself and immediately both Ivan and I relaxed. Gradually more and more relatives arrived to greet Ivan and me. Everyone was kind, warm, and welcoming. Any preconceived ideas that I had washed away as I got to talk with them and spend time with them over the next few days. I felt right at home with his relatives.

Ivan's family had rented a tux for him. He was even included in the ceremony as a candle lighter. He looked so handsome in his tux. I was used to seeing him with baggy jeans that hung off his butt showing several inches of underwear, along with oversized shirts, and high top tennis shoes. Though Ivan wasn't excited about being dressed in such formal clothes, I liked this new look.

The day after the wedding the family treated us like special guests and took us around San Francisco, including lunch at a nice restaurant built on a cliff overlooking the ocean. They treated me like I was already Ivan's mom. I came away feeling like I knew his family and they knew me. In the future when he talked about his relatives, they were more than just names to me. I knew what they looked like and what their personalities were like. I had a connection with them. It was a valuable trip.

Ivan didn't want to leave, and in some ways neither did I. Spending those days helped me to also have some understanding as to why none of the relatives had stepped forward, for a variety of reasons, to rescue Ivan out of the foster care system and raise him themselves. It can be easy to pass judgment when you don't have all the information. I went away knowing that it wasn't a lack of love that kept Ivan's extended family from intervening in his life. I shared with his family they were welcome to come and visit Ivan any time they could travel to Washington. Like I told Seneca, we wanted to add to Ivan's life, not take away from it. His relatives, though separated from him by distance, still loved Ivan and he still loved them.

Cindy Locke

CHAPTER 6

Two weeks after we returned home from
California, we had a large family birthday party for
Josiah. At his party we were able to announce our plan
to adopt Ivan. Most of our extended family already knew
and loved Ivan and were excited for us. A few though
still couldn't figure out why we would want to adopt a
16 year old.

When the party started winding down, my niece
Leah and her husband Phil approached us. They shared
that they wanted to take Ivan and Jordan on a trip to

Hawaii. Ivan had received his laptop computer and iPod from the Make a Wish Foundation, but Phil wanted him to have a special trip also. Phil and Leah were planning to go in the summer and were hoping to bring the boys along. They said that they would pay for the trip and had connections to get some of it donated, including a luxury condominium in Maui. Both Jordan and Ivan were excited and began dreaming what they could do in Hawaii. I was hoping that the adoption would be completed by that time. Having foster children fly out of state, especially with a person other than the foster parent, is difficult to get approved. If Ivan was adopted, all those issues would be nonexistent.

Three months had passed since Ivan's last scans, but now it was time again for him to get checked. Just like the past two times, my anxiety rose a few days before the appointment. Ivan seemed so healthy and alive that I tried to assure myself that everything was fine. Whenever I would tell Ivan I was nervous about the scans, he'd let me know I was being ridiculous. He certainly wasn't nervous.

I knew the ropes this time. We went to multiple scans in the morning, a several hour long lunch break, then returned to the clinic to get the results.

During this lunch break Ivan asked if we could go driving around the University of Washington campus. He wasn't in pursuit of education; he wanted to check out any "hot" girls that may be out and about. I thought why not, a trip to the nearby campus would pass the time more quickly. What a ridiculous trip. Some middle age mom driving her 16 year old son around so he could check out the girls. Ivan was unique. He would tell me exactly what he liked and didn't like in girls, including what he liked in their body shape. He especially didn't like what he called pancake butt. Now most teenage boys might think like this, but there aren't many who would tell their mom these things! I tried to instill some morals into the situation when he started ogling over an especially curvaceous young woman's hind end.

"Butts are for padding". I informed him.

Ivan, "Butts are for patting?"

"No, butts are for padding!" I corrected.

"Butts are for petting?" he said with a twinkle in his eye and a smirk on his face. Silly Ivan, typical sixteen, I loved this boy and I loved that he let me in to his world.

After our "scenic" drive, we returned to the hospital for the results. I was nervous, but didn't really think we were going to hear anything except, "all the scans are clear," like we had heard the past two times. We were taken to an exam room we'd visited many times before. Sue, the nurse practitioner, soon joined us. With a matter of fact expression, Sue announced that Ivan's CT scan showed 5-8 nodules in his lungs. They weren't 100% sure that this was the return of the cancer, but for now they were assuming that it was. I was shocked and felt numb. Whenever I looked over at Ivan he would look me in the eyes and smile. I guess you always wonder how you would feel and react if you ever got this type of news. This was not the reaction I would have expected from me or Ivan. I felt nothing but numbness, like my emotions had been shut off, and all Ivan could do was smile. I knew that if they were right, this meant we were just told that Ivan would die. The boy I loved so deeply was dying, yet I couldn't feel anything. I was in shock. Very little else was said as we processed the news in our different ways.

The car ride home was quiet. Occasionally I'd

glance over at Ivan and he would say, "You look so sad." or, "You look like you are about to cry." He however was still smiling or staring out the window.

The plan was for him to return in 6 weeks to see if the nodules had grown. If they did grow we would know for certain it was cancer. Ivan stated that he wouldn't believe the cancer was back until they proved to him that the nodules had grown. He would carry on like nothing had changed and believe he was fine.

The emotional numbness wore off by the next day. Waves of tears and sadness overwhelmed me. If he was with me, bouncing around, happy and full of life, I was fine. When he wasn't around, the pain was debilitating. We tried to get back to normal living as best we could.

A few days after the scans I went outside and I saw a large green mucous plug that someone had coughed up and spit on the driveway. My mind immediately thought that it must be from Ivan. That must have been what they saw on the scan. He is ok I rationalized, all they saw was an infection. My mind was trying to find anything to combat the fear that I felt. In light of all the emotions that were surfacing I found it complicated to know how to parent Ivan. This wasn't covered in parenting 101. The rest of the kids knew that they needed to come home and get their homework done. They'd had the same routines since they were in kindergarten. My goal was for them to grow up to be responsible people who could hold down a job and make a difference in the world. What about Ivan? What am I supposed to do when he comes home from school and plops down on the couch and starts to play the Wii, or gets up in the morning and decides he doesn't want to go to school that day? Does it matter if he even does his homework? Does it even matter if he goes to school? If he is truly dying, does any of that matter? No one gave me a manual on parenting a teenager who in all likelihood was dying. Ivan and I would just have to figure this out together.

There were questions now about the adoption. Jami, Lenny, and I began to discuss what we should do next. Fear began to creep in, how will we afford to pay for an adoption and a funeral back to back? What if the insurance doesn't cover all of his medical bills? I was afraid that if we followed through and adopted Ivan, that just when he needed me to care for him 24 hours a day, I might need to go back to work to support him. Would it just be safer to stick with foster care and not have to worry about the financial part? Eventually, we all agreed that now more than ever Ivan needed a forever family, and we needed Ivan. We decided we were willing to take the risk, and asked Jami if she could try to speed up the adoption.

The biggest road block was getting the approval from Ivan's tribe. Nothing could happen until we had their permission. Jami immediately wrote a letter to the tribe and explained the situation. She faxed it to them and miraculously, within 24 hours, they had signed and returned the paperwork! From what I've been told, this never happens. The biggest obstacle we saw in the adoption process was suddenly complete. It gave us hope.

The next step was to get our home study updated. Darby, the caseworker, who sent us the notice about Ivan, made us a priority. The State of Alaska and our foster care agency were in discussion about who would pay for the updated home study, our family, or the State of Alaska. Darby said she would do the home study and worry about payment later. We quickly filled out all the paperwork and made the appointment for our home inspection and interview portion. Darby knew our family well and was able to update our prior home study quickly.

The next 6 weeks crept slowly by as we waited to go in to have Ivan's lungs rescanned. Some days I was so confident that all they saw on the scan was an infection, and at other times I was convinced that the cancer was back. I had wild emotional swings. There were moments of pure grief to be sure, but there were also moments of pure joy, when watching Ivan with all his exuberance for life. There was excitement that the adoption was getting closer along with a sense of terror in finding out the true meaning of the last scans.

In the midst of all this I decided to search on the internet for Travis, the young man that also had Ewing's Sarcoma. The last time I had seen him at the hospital he was looking weak and pale, being pushed in a wheelchair by his mom. This was in direct contrast to the first time I'd recognized him at the hospital, when he'd driven himself and looked like a healthy teenage boy. I found a follow up story that was run about him in the local paper, now posted to the internet. He had recently passed away. I was so afraid that Ivan was on

the same path, just a few months behind Travis. I
prayed daily that God would grant us a miracle like he
gave to our friends John and Susan for baby Brent. I
knew God was able to heal him, I'd seen Brent recover
from a hopeless state to full health. At times I prayed
boldly for Ivan's healing, at other times I was almost
afraid to hope.

The time finally came to find out the truth of
what was happening inside Ivan's body. I wasn't as
nervous as the last scans. As far as I saw it, they could
only give us good news since they previously had given
us the bad news 6 weeks ago. As we drove down to the
hospital I thought about the recent shooting at the
Virginia Tech College, where a gunman had killed 32
people. I thought of all the families who never got to say
goodbye, never got to hug their loved ones just one more
time. At least if the cancer was back, we would get to
say goodbye and pour out our love on Ivan. Those
families would never have that chance.

We went in for the CT scan and found out that
the nodules were indeed tumors, and that they were
growing. Sue pulled the images up on a computer screen
and we were face to face with the monster. It was

undeniable, we could see the tumors plain and clear. As we expected there wasn't much that could be done. An open chest biopsy could be performed to confirm that this was cancer. There were also research "trials" that were being carried out, but Sue didn't think Ivan would qualify for them. Beyond him not qualifying, I also knew that Ivan would not consent to more chemotherapy. His year of surgery and chemo was still too fresh, and he did not want to repeat it. I was sure he wouldn't want to be opened up just to prove it was cancer. Instead, he would be switched to palliative care, medical intervention to keep him comfortable, not treatments to try and cure the cancer. When the time came he would get hospice care in our home.

I asked Sue, "Does Ivan have weeks, months, or years left?"

"Months." was Sue's reply.

Ivan and I behaved similarly to this appointment as we had 6 weeks earlier. I went numb and he just smiled at me. What are you supposed to do after you are told you are dying? Ivan and I went to Taco Bell and picked up lunch.

As we sat in the car I asked him, "So now what?"

He said "I just want to keep living until I die."

His words were simple yet honest. He didn't want to lay around feeling sorry for himself; he had too much living to get done. So that was the new plan, get as much living in as possible.

Later that same day I got a call from my mom. My dad had gone in for some medical tests himself. The reports came back and he was diagnosed with an aggressive form of prostate cancer. My mind was already so full of grief, I could not handle anymore coming in. My emotions numbed again. After dinner, Lenny and I sat the kids down, while Ivan was busy in his room, to tell them the news. Not only was their brother told that the cancer was back and his life was going to be cut short, their grandfather was also diagnosed with cancer. There's no way to sugar coat either diagnosis, cancer in any form is life changing. Now we had two family members confronting different cancers at the same time. The kids were stunned and quiet, except for Sarah, who burst out crying while she was alone with Lenny. She had a special closeness with

Ivan and the grief she felt was instantaneous and overwhelming.

I had called my niece Leah, and her husband Phil after the appointment. That evening they came over to the house. As we talked, I expressed my concern about whether or not Ivan would be healthy enough to go to Hawaii in the summer. It was now April. I had asked Sue if she felt by summer he would still be strong enough for a big trip. She said he might be just the same as he is now, or he might be a lot weaker; cancer is so unpredictable. I wanted him to be able to go and enjoy Hawaii. Phil said he would start working on getting everything set up. Since they weren't going to wait until summer, this meant that Leah and Jordan wouldn't be able to go with them. Jordan couldn't afford to miss a week of school and Leah was a teacher and couldn't take the time off with such short notice. I was sad for Jordan, he had been looking forward to the trip just as much as Ivan. But Jordan, the emotionally level person that he is, never once complained about the change in plans. Phil and Ivan would now be going alone, if the State of Alaska would approve it.

Since we weren't able to finalize the adoption

first, we were going to have to cut through both states red tape. Within days Phil got plane tickets for the end of April. An acquaintance of his had a luxury condominium in Maui that he set 8 days aside for the two of them to stay in while there. Friends and co-workers donated money for them to go on excursions and for food while in Hawaii. Ivan was getting excited to have a "guy's trip" to Hawaii. Phil was young and though newly married, I'm sure Ivan had ideas of the two of them following "hot" chicks around on the beaches. Just two dudes, sun, sand, and bikini clad young women was all Ivan could think about. Living was his plan and he was going to get some "living" in.

Everything was coming together except permission from the state of Alaska for Ivan to travel with Phil. This was very short notice for them, and they were saying that Phil needed a criminal history check and finger prints before he left the state with Ivan. I knew that finger prints took several weeks, if not months to process. My anxiety began increasing as the time got closer for them to leave. I started to make a backup plan. I would just buy my own plane ticket and go along if they couldn't get it approved for Phil to take him. In my mind, this was the best solution. Ivan would still be able to go and I'd give them space. I could hang out at the condo or enjoy the nearby beach while they did their own thing.

I told Ivan about my wonderful back up plan. He said that if I went he didn't want to go. WHAT???? I was furious and hurt. I was doing this so that he could go, and he had the nerve to tell me this. I was so upset that I took off for a long walk. I walked to a friend's house and as I entered I said "I want to kill the dying boy!" I shared what just happened and then took off walking again. When I returned I went to his room and told him that I thought he was ungrateful and mean spirited, and that his comment hurt my feelings. After unloading on him I left him in his room.

A postal truck arrived shortly after my verbal assault. Jami had sent a box of his records. This was part of the preparation for Ivan's adoption. The state was mandated to release the records to us so that we would know what he'd been through and the issues we might face raising him. We needed to read the files, so that later we couldn't sue the state for withholding information from us. I took the files to my room and sat on my bed reading his history. I had been told some of it, but as I read through volumes of records documenting his life, I realized how far he had come both medically and emotionally. The years in residential treatment and psychiatric facilities, his suicide attempts, the abandonment he endured from his father; all was laid out before me.

Intertwined in Ivan's story was Seneca's story. As I read about Ivan, I understood more about Seneca. We had not seen Seneca since Thanksgiving. He had only stayed in contact with Ivan by phone calls and text. I had occasionally spoken to him on the phone, but not seen him. This is not how I wanted everything to unfold. I had always imagined Seneca being a very big part of Ivan's life in our home. I still wasn't sure why he had pulled away. Ivan and I had called him about the cancer returning. I wondered how he was processing the news. I could only imagine that he was hurting as bad, or worse than me. After reading the reports I felt I had a better understanding of Seneca. Reading the files helped me unwind and get the focus off myself. I started to see that Ivan just wanted to go to Hawaii, be the handsome 16 year old guy on the beach with Phil, his 20 something side kick. He didn't want his Mommy hanging around. I understood that.

Ivan had gone from an introverted boy who hung on me like a little child, to a young man who needed his space from his mother, all in less than a year. The change was so rapid it was hard to keep up with. I calmed down by the time I'd read several of the reports. I just wanted Ivan to have a good time in Hawaii, however that happened. When I entered his room later he said "I never meant to hurt you". I could tell in his eyes he was sincere. I assured him that I understood that he just wanted to be a teenage boy on the beach without his mommy hanging around. We would do our best to get him there without me. We hugged and the whole emotional explosion was over.

A few days later, and just days before their departure date, the State of Alaska approved Phil taking Ivan to Hawaii. The State of Alaska had received a copy of the finger print clearance that Phil had completed for his current job as a loan officer. I was happy that Ivan was going. However, even 8 days away from him seemed like it would be too long knowing his life was going to be cut short.

Ivan was so excited once the approval came in. He was feeling as physically strong as he had felt since the cancer was diagnosed. Internally he was settled and free. Around the house he was full of pranks and fun. There was never a dull moment when Ivan was around. A few days before he was supposed to leave to go to Hawaii, Ivan was pretending to karate kick Jordan, who was sitting on the couch watching television. Instead of hitting the air, or Jordan's face, he kicked the couch. He immediately stopped and hobbled to the nearest place to sit. I got ice as we watched his foot begin to swell. He wouldn't admit to how bad it hurt and said he was fine as he half hopped and limped back to his room to go to bed. He called me a whiner for making such a big deal about it. By the next morning Ivan was no longer able to walk on his foot. He still had not been back to the hospital since his scans and refused to go in to have it looked at by a physician. But with Hawaii coming in a couple days, and my incessant nagging, he finally agreed to have it checked.

I put a call into his nurse practitioner and explained what happened. She made arrangements for him to go straight to the x-ray department, without getting an exam first, to minimize the time and emotional discomfort of being in a hospital. She then arranged for an orthopedic doctor to see him immediately after the x-ray. I had no crutches at home for him to use to get into the hospital, so I told Ivan I would bring his wheelchair for this appointment.

"I won't get in a wheelchair." He replied.

"Are you going to hop all the way into the hospital?" I asked.

"Yes. No wheelchair!" So he hopped all the way to the car and got in.

At least he agreed to go; if he wanted to hop the whole way, I guess that was his choice. We arrived and I parked as close as I could, but it was still a distance to get into the hospital, let alone to the x-ray department. Ivan took off hoping on one foot, before long he was holding onto my shoulder and then I was practically carrying him. "Ivan, this is ridiculous! Just get in a wheelchair. No one will care, it isn't like you are paralyzed again, you probably broke your foot." We made it to the automatic doors of the hospital and saw a collection of wheelchairs waiting. Ivan finally climbed into one and off we went. Without a hitch we whizzed through the x-ray and saw the doctor. His foot was broken and he was given a removable walking cast.

Needless to say, this was not the best time for him to break his foot. At least he didn't have a fiberglass type cast that would have prevented him from swimming. We were hopeful the pain would diminish a bit before he arrived in Hawaii so he could still enjoy his time there.

The next couple of days Ivan rested and kept his foot elevated. By the time Phil came to pick him up the morning of the trip, Ivan was getting around pretty well in his walking cast. Phil had done all the work to get most of the trip, condo, food and adventures donated. I was so thankful for all Phil and others had done to provide this experience for Ivan. As a nervous mom I put together a folder of Ivan's medical information including the latest x-ray of his broken foot, and all the contact information for his doctors and caseworkers. I was praying that nothing more would go wrong while he was nearly 3000 miles away and out of my care.

I hugged him and the two of them headed off on their big adventure. The other kids were at school. Alone in the house, I crawled into my bed and wept for what seemed like hours. Though he was just gone to Hawaii, and only for 8 days, my mind and body felt like he was gone for good. Someday I would be apart from him and he would not be coming back. At times the grief was like someone was sitting on my chest and I couldn't catch my breath. I literally felt like I couldn't breathe. I had heard of debilitating grief, and had felt a little bit of it when my grandfather and my friend Joyce died, but never had I felt it to the point I couldn't function, couldn't breathe, couldn't cope. My love for this boy was crazy. It was as deep as my love and attachment for any of my other children, and the pain from the thought of losing him was immobilizing.

A friend called to check in on me. She could tell I wasn't coping well. Soon a team of people had been rallied to prepare and bring meals. Receiving several meals, along with the love and support of dear friends over the next several days, went a long way to show that we were loved and not alone on this journey. Each day, as the time grew near for the kids to arrive home from school, I would try to pull myself together and become the mom they knew. They weren't sure why meals were being brought for our family, but ate them happily anyways.

Several days into the trip Phil called to give me an update. The two of them were having fun, but Ivan was still quite shy and not talking a whole lot. Even at home, Ivan would still retreat into his nearly non-verbal self when he was with people outside of our circle of close family members.

Ivan had been refusing to wear his walking cast unless it benefitted him, such as when he was able to pre-board the plane because of his injury. Except for times like that, his walking cast was thrown aside, and he chose to hobble on his broken foot. On the plus side, he'd had an awesome experience swimming with a sea turtle. Then Phil told me a funny story that helped the grief lift for a little while. Ivan had heard about the nude beaches in the area and was determined to go to one. Phil told him that he would take him, but told him not to expect much. The two guys had made their way from the parking area along a trail leading to the beach, Ivan hobbling on his broken foot without the support of the walking cast. I imagined that Ivan's endurance was likely motivated by visions of naked Hawaiian beauties lounging along the beach. As they neared their destination they crested a hill heading to the beach where the beauties awaited him. There, directly in front of them, was the backside of a large, naked, hairy man. Ivan stated, "I think I've had enough of the nude beach!"

turned and hobbled back to the car. During the remainder of the time he was in Hawaii, that story bounced around in my mind making me chuckle, protecting me a little from the waves of grief that continued to roll through my soul.

CHAPTER 7

Once Ivan returned home from Hawaii he made
the decision not to go back to school. I had spoken with
Sue regarding the whole idea of him stopping school
versus continuing. She counseled me that there was no
clear cut answer. If the child enjoys school and wants to
go then great, if he wants to stay home then that is fine
too. A lot of kids miss their routine and their friends
from school, so it is better for them to go. Ivan just
wanted to stay home. It was strange to not have the
pressure to force him to go, no one from the school was

calling and threatening with enforcement of the BECA bill, a bill passed to keep kids from skipping school.

The teachers told me that he could come when he wanted, and stay home when he wanted. There would be no pressure to keep up with homework or assignments; he could attend just for the social aspect of school. He chose to stay home. He was healthy and strong, and right then he did not look sick. I continued to make him get up at a reasonable hour and he would run errands with me or hang out around the house playing video games.

Occasionally our youth pastor, Phil would come pick Ivan up and take him places, or come and visit with him for a while. Ivan had only attended church with us a couple of times. He was very uncomfortable in the building but he liked the people. Pastor Phil and several of the young adults and teens formed relationships with him outside of the church walls in an environment that Ivan was comfortable in. One day Pastor Phil picked up Ivan to run errands. On their outing they stopped by the workplace of one of the young adults from our church. His name is Eryk, and he was a Porsche mechanic. That day it just so happened that he needed to take a car for a test drive. Eryk invited Ivan along in the two seat sports car. Ivan was so excited to tell me about it when he got home. I was excited for him also, until he informed me that they had topped 120 mph on the freeway. After a stern scolding, Eryk and I became friends and his name was changed to Bad Boy Eryk. Encounters like the one with Eryk brought people into Ivan's life. There was something special about Ivan, once people met him they tended to stay connected with him.

The kids started rolling in a little bit after 2pm every day, so he always had plenty of teenagers to do things with in the afternoon and evenings. Ivan loved hanging out with the kids, but I also knew he was missing Seneca. Their communication via text and phone calls had picked up since we told Seneca that the cancer had returned in mid-April. Even though we rarely had contact with Seneca, I still worried about him. I still couldn't figure out why, after being so devoted to Ivan for the entire year that he was in cancer treatment that he seemed to have vanished. I knew the brothers loved each other and I knew Ivan wanted to see Seneca much more often. It was now getting towards the end of May, I needed to pursue Seneca.

In just a few more weeks the adoption was scheduled to take place and Seneca still didn't even know that we were adopting him. Ivan and I encouraged Seneca to come up for the day to hang out with us. Seneca agreed, and took the bus to a nearby transit center where Ivan and I met him. It had been 6 months since we had seen him. I hardly recognized him because his hair was noticeably longer. The ride back to the house was slightly awkward for me. I wasn't sure if I should be mad that Seneca had seemingly dropped out of Ivan's life for the past 6 months, or sad for all he had been going through. I did realize that there had to be more to his story. Though I was upset by Seneca's absence, the brothers didn't seem to have any distance between them when they were reunited.

Back at the house they hung out in Ivan's room catching up with each other. I had asked Ivan to make sure that he told Seneca about the adoption during their time together. Later in the evening I poked my head into Ivan's room. I could tell that Seneca had heard about the adoption. To be sure, I asked Seneca if Ivan had told him. He nodded, and by his body language I could tell it was a painful blow.

That evening after dinner, and after the brothers had a few hours to be together, I made an excuse as to why Ivan needed to stay home. I wanted to take Seneca back to his apartment by myself so I could find out how he was doing with all the news. There was a lot to discuss, Ivan's cancer returning and our family adopting his brother were both huge issues affecting not only our family but even more so Seneca in many ways.

Like Ivan, Seneca and I communicated well in the car. He told me about the pain of hearing that the cancer had come back. How he had only his girlfriend to share his sadness with. The adoption was a second blow. I could tell he feared that we were going to take his brother away from him. He had been kept from Ivan before. He was convinced the same thing would happen again. I assured him that we wanted him to be a part of Ivan's life. We wanted to add to his life, not take anyone out of his life. I felt so sorry for Seneca. My heart broke for him. He still didn't believe us when we said that we cared for him too.

After talking about these sensitive and painful topics in the parking lot, I got out of the car to hug him good bye. I hugged him for a very long time. He and

Ivan were similar in so many ways. He was more melancholy and quiet, compared to Ivan's silliness, but both of them had such kind and sensitive hearts. I told him the date that was scheduled for the adoption and encouraged him to come with us. The plan was for his grandma and his cousin, to come up from California to also attend. I was hoping that Seneca would come too, if not to celebrate the adoption, then to at least be able to see them. He said he would see about coming, but wasn't sure if he could get off of work. I knew this was an excuse, he had told me earlier that the tattoo shop that he recently began working at was new and didn't receive much business.

The next day I wrote him a long letter and sent some money along for his upcoming birthday. I reiterated that we wanted to walk with him through this painful time. I felt strongly that it would benefit all of us, Ivan, Seneca, and our family, if we went through this season together. We needed each other now, and I knew we would need each other even more as Ivan's health deteriorated. I hoped he would feel our sincerity and whatever was holding him back from being involved in Ivan's and our family's lives, would go away.

June was busy getting the last minute legal paperwork completed for the adoption. By this point most of the anxiety around adopting Ivan had faded away. In my heart he was already my son. We just needed the paperwork to make it official.

Ivan's grandma and cousin came the day before the adoption. I had gotten to know each of them a bit at the California wedding, but to the rest of the family they were new. They fit right in and Ivan's cousin, 13 at the time, got along with all the kids right off. Ivan was able to reach Seneca, and between the both of us, we convinced him to come with us the following day.

The next day we loaded our 12 passenger van with our whole family, along with Ivan's grandma and cousin, and went to pick up Seneca at the tattoo shop where he was working. We were all in a happy, excited mood as we picked him up. Seneca seemed more like he was going to a funeral and remained subdued and quiet, though he did chat with his grandma and cousin.

Ivan's social worker, Jami, and Ivan's guardian ad litem, Bobby, had flown down from Alaska to be present at the adoption. Both of them had invested so much into Ivan, and had walked the hard road with him

141

over the past several years. I felt honored to have them attend. My parents, and my brother and his family also met us at the court house.

The actual ceremony was short. The judge asked Lenny, myself, and Ivan questions about our intent to become a family, with all the rights and responsibilities that are included in being parents and a son. We all stated "I do" like we were getting married. The judge had read the court reports and knew Ivan's story. He made some comments about how great it was for us to adopt Ivan with all that he was going through. To me, I was the blessed one. To adopt a teenage boy that was so full of love and life was a huge blessing. The way that Ivan allowed himself to love us, and allowed us to love him back was my greatest joy. People often think that adoptive families are giving, and the adopted child is receiving, but we were receiving as much as Ivan. He was our gift and our family felt honored to be able to call him our son and brother.

After the ceremony and pictures with the judge, we all headed back to our house for an adoption party. Friends joined us there as we celebrated the adoption. Lenny and I had made a slide show put to music to show at the party. Jami cried while watching it, but Ivan was embarrassed because we put a couple pictures of him in while he was still bald from his chemo. Seneca still seemed somewhat subdued as the party atmosphere continued.

I hated seeing Seneca so sad when everyone else was laughing and having a good time. Finally I asked Seneca to go outside with me. On the corner of the deck, out of everyone's view, I talked again about how adopting Ivan was not about cutting him out of Ivan's life, we wanted to be family to him also. I told him that the kids had asked, "If Ivan and Seneca are brothers and we adopt Ivan does that make Seneca our brother also?" I told them that "Yes, it kind of makes Seneca a brother also." They were so excited about that.

He asked. "Did they really say that?"

"Yes, they really said that." I assured him.

Seneca broke down crying, I hugged him as he sobbed. Maybe, just maybe, he would believe me now. Maybe he would allow us to love him too.

Cindy Locke

CHAPTER 8

The adoption was now over and summer had begun. The kids were out of school and Ivan was officially part of the family. Though we loved Jami, we were so happy to make decisions without having to consult her or wait for the state of Alaska to give us permission to do things. Ivan was no longer a "foster child," he was a brother and son.

Ivan was healthy, happy, and always full of pranks. With no more appointments at the hospital and him being strong and healthy, it was easy to just forget about the cancer. It was no longer in the fore front of our minds. Having fun, going camping, and just being a family was the main thing we were focusing on doing that summer. The intense grief of the Spring had subsided. We were all just enjoying life.

We had originally wanted to take the family to Yellowstone that year. However, when it was time to reserve campsites and make plans, we were afraid to be so far from home in case Ivan began getting sick. We opted instead to go camping on the Olympic Peninsula. We camped on the ocean beach for the first few days. The kids were in their element and the weather was perfect. Jordan and Ivan created driftwood bridges across freshwater streams, as the other kids made sand castles and searched for creatures. Ivan was always pushing the boundaries of safety. Unlike my other kids who have a more conservative nature, Ivan needed a bit of adrenaline now and then. While exploring the beach he found a tree that was growing on the side of a cliff, half of its roots were exposed and hanging down. The tree was leaning out over the beach appearing like it could let go at any time. With jagged rocks below, it looked like it could have been a prop for the show Fear Factor. Of course, this was just the tree Ivan wanted to climb. Part of me said, just let him climb and explore.

The other part of me said, you may be dying but I don't want it to be from falling out of a tree onto jagged rocks! I battled in my mind until I couldn't handle watching him anymore. "Ivan get down before you fall out of that tree and kill yourself. You may be dying but we don't want it to happen now." He reluctantly climbed down from the tree. I was always the one to ruin his fun. With not much of a pause, he was off to find a new adventure. A year before he could barely climb a flight of stairs, now his body could take him anywhere his mind wanted to go. The joy I felt as I watched him run and climb and be free in his body was amazing.

Emotionally he was free also. At one campsite we were sitting around one evening making s'mores at the camp fire. We heard someone on the other side of some trees yell "Does anyone have a can opener?" The whole family except Ivan sat there trying to figure out what was happening.

Ivan instantly yelled "I do!"

The unknown people yelled back "Can we borrow it?"

Ivan yelled "Yes," and then walked the can

opener over to them.

For the next hour or so Ivan and the young adults on the other side yelled back and forth to each other through the trees as they thought of other things they had forgotten. Then it turned into random words that they would shout to each other. One side would yell "coconut" and the other would yell "pineapple." While Ivan and the other group yelled back and forth, the rest of our family sat around the campfire and chuckled at the whole thing. Ivan could create fun out of the mundane and he didn't care about standard protocol. Every day was an adventure with Ivan. Boring moments never stayed that way for long as he would always break up the monotony with something unexpected.

After our family trip to the coast we were back home for a few weeks. Ivan had met a family while staying at the Ronald McDonald house during the year he lived there. Even though Ivan hadn't been much of a talker back then, Seneca, Ivan and the Carroll family had formed a relationship. The Carroll family was from Montana and stayed in Seattle while their eleven year old son, Caleb, was treated for Leukemia. Sheila, Caleb's mom, had become very fond of both Seneca and

Ivan. We had remained in contact over the year by phone and had met up with them a couple times when Caleb had been in Seattle for checkups. Sheila had invited Ivan to come to Montana to spend a week with them. Besides Caleb, they also had a teenage daughter that I think Ivan was looking forward to getting to know better. I was so glad that we didn't have to get permission to do this sort of outing anymore. I trusted Ivan, and I trusted the Carroll family, and that was all I needed. No caseworker or judge had to sign off on the trip. Ivan had stated his goal was to get as much living in as possible. This was living to Ivan. So with his packed bag and cell phone I dropped him off at the Greyhound station. The experience was so much different than when he went to Hawaii. Maybe because I was in denial at that point, or maybe because the kids were home for the summer, whatever the reason I didn't cry the week he was away. I was excited for Ivan and happy that he got a chance to go on an adventure by himself.

When he returned he had plenty of stories to tell of things he did in Montana. He told us about joining a make believe "family" on the 22 hour bus ride where he was one of the "kids." Random people who had been traveling alone joined together and became a family. The boy who didn't speak or make eye contact not very long ago was now making friends and joining groups in just hours.

Still wanting to believe a miracle had happened, but also wanting to be prepared ahead of time, so I could focus on Ivan if he began getting sick, I went to the funeral home. I had to go over to the cemetery a couple of times. I'd give Ivan the excuse that I was running errands or something, so that he didn't know what I was actually doing. It was really surreal making funeral arrangements for my teenage son, who appeared just about as healthy as any 16 year old boy. Sue, his nurse practitioner, had said he only had months to live, and 4 months had already passed. I wasn't sure how fast he would become sick, and I didn't want to be spending that time dealing with arrangements.

One day I returned from grocery shopping and Ivan said "The funeral home called for you".

Great, what do you say to that? "Ok. Do you have any questions?" I asked Ivan.

"Nope, I'm good." he replied.

I put away the groceries then went to a different

room and called the funeral home back. "Don't ever call my house again and say that it is the funeral home. You just left a message with my teenage son who is dying, and he doesn't need to be dealing with this!" I was livid and not very kind on the phone. From then on they sent me e-mails.

Cindy Locke

CHAPTER 9

Labor Day weekend came. Our beautiful fun filled summer was coming to an end. Ivan had been healthy all summer. No signs of cancer, no apparent weight loss… maybe a miracle had occurred. The entire family spent Labor Day working in the yard, putting away our large swimming pool, and getting ready for fall and winter. Ivan, along with Jordan, was busy cutting and hauling the black berry brambles that had snuck into our yard. The weather was warm and pleasant for working outside.

When we were nearly finished, Ivan and I snuck

away to get slurpees for the entire family. He still loved going places with me, even on boring shopping trips, and I always loved having his company. It continued to be where we had our best conversations. I think it was less threatening in the car because we didn't have to make eye contact and there wasn't a chance the other kids would come walking in, right in the middle of a personal conversation. Today he was my helper, since I knew I couldn't carry eight slurpees on my own. We arrived back with the treats and all sat around in the yard. Our 2/3rds acre yard was beautiful when it was mowed, weeded, and all trimmed up. As a family we had worked hard for several hours, now we could just enjoy being together and feel like we'd accomplished something. In the back of my mind I was eager to get this chore taken care of before the weather changed. I wasn't sure when Ivan's symptoms would begin, and I knew when they did that it would be the only thing our family would be able to focus on. Yard work would not be a priority, neither would most anything else.

The next day school began. Like most years, there was a happy/ sad feeling for the kids going back to school. The kids were excited to get back to class to see their friends, yet not wanting to give up the fun and carefree days of the summer.

Ivan had decided he now wanted to go back to school full time. He hadn't been to school since April, and since his health was still good, he needed the social outlet. Ivan had been communicating with a girl on a social networking site and was looking forward to meeting her in person at school. It was odd for me to have the house quiet again all day, and I didn't especially like it. Except for occasionally checking on my Grandma Rose in her studio apartment, I was left to just clean the house, grocery shop, and get ready for all the kids returning home in the afternoon. It was somewhat boring for my liking.

The following weekend our family, and my parents, were invited by a friend of theirs to go to his family's lake house, an hour drive north of us. Rich, my parent's friend, had heard about Ivan's struggle with cancer and was well aware of the difficulties my dad was having with his own cancer treatments. We were to stay both Friday and Saturday nights. Rich was planning the meals and bringing all the food, we were instructed to just pack our clothes and come. We were all looking forward to this weekend. We had seen pictures of the house, which looked more like a mansion than a cabin on a lake. They had a ski boat, kayaks, and a private dock for fishing. Rich's son, Brian, had planned to join us with his kids on Saturday to drive the ski boat and teach our kids how to wakeboard. We felt honored to have been invited by them.

Friday I noticed Ivan had a little bit of a cough. I wasn't too concerned about it though because Jordan had a cold of his own that first week of school. Often times the kids get sick in September when they all rejoin the hundreds of other kids back at school. Lenny got off from work a couple hours early so we could get a jump on our weekend adventure. We all piled into our 12 passenger van and headed north on Interstate 5.

We arrived at the lake house about dinner time. The house was bigger and even more beautiful than the pictures. I was almost afraid to let my six kids loose in such a beautiful home. Rich, a friendly man with a big smile, met us in the driveway and greeted us. He showed us around the house and the property and explained that there was one house rule, and that was to make ourselves feel at home.

My parents arrived a short time later. My dad,

weak from 40 rounds of radiation, headed to the big leather recliner chair in the living room. All of us claimed different rooms in the house and stowed our belongings. Jordan, Ivan, and Josiah took a large apartment that was built over the huge detached garage. The rest of us had rooms in the main house. When we were all moved in, we gathered in the large dining room and ate lasagna dinner that Rich had prepared for us. The view from the dining room was breath taking. We looked out over the deck, across the lawn, and past the private dock to a beautiful lake. Different types of water fowl swam about, and great blue heron were often seen resting and sunning themselves on the dock. After dinner the kids found themselves down at the dock, lying on their bellies watching the fish swim about in the waters below. The temperature was warm even as the sun began to set. We were all so happy to be together.

The next morning Lenny and I awoke to the smell of bacon and waffles. I could hear the kids downstairs helping Rich make the breakfast. Soon Sarah and Kailey arrived with our breakfast. Sitting with Lenny in our luxurious suite looking over the lake with a layer of mist sitting on the surface of the water and eating our wonderful breakfast, we felt like royalty.

There was a feeling of gratitude not for just being spoiled for the weekend, but a deeper sense of gratitude for belonging to this family. I felt extremely grateful to have a family who really loved each other and liked spending time together. Having three teenagers who liked hanging out with their parents was definitely something rare and we were so grateful.

Ivan was not part of the early morning cooking crew since he still was not an early riser. He found his way to breakfast about the time the rest of us were finishing up. His cough was still bothering him. It was a deep cough, yet still fairly infrequent and not productive. Jordan's cough was starting to taper off, so I hoped Ivan's would also.

The plan was for Brian, Rich's son, to arrive mid-morning to get the ski boat out of the garage and put it in the lake. After breakfast Ivan, Kailey, and I headed down to the lake and put the kayaks in the water. They had a two person kayak and a one person kayak. After putting on life jackets we headed out on the lake. Ivan was in the single boat, and Kailey and I in the double. It was a beautiful morning. The fog had lifted from the water and the bright blue sky was beautiful. There was a peaceful quiet in the morning, before all the ski boats and jet skis were out. Various ducks and other colorful water fowl paddled about on the water. We didn't seem to bother them unless we got within a few feet, then they would just paddle off in another direction and leave us behind.

Ivan was still much stronger than Kailey and I combined. We attempted to chase him but it was a futile attempt. He would take off across the water in the green kayak and just laugh at our attempts to outrun him. Ivan looked so happy and healthy. His collar-length-light brown-wavy hair, along with his summer time tan and lightly freckled cheeks, made him a handsome teenager. His eyes were bright and his smile was now real and full. No more keeping his teeth covered as he put on a pretend smile like last year. Ivan was fully alive and fully part of our family.

After a half hour of playing in the kayaks we headed back to the dock. The rest of the kids had found the fishing poles and were now happily attempting to bait their hooks to catch the fish they could see swimming in and around the dock. Ivan and Kailey joined them preparing their poles and hooks. Before long all six kids were laying on their bellies in the sunshine waiting to catch the "big one." I joined them just to watch and be part of the experience. It was magical and I would have chosen that dock over anywhere else in the whole world.

Before long Brian showed up and introductions were made. He and Lenny used our van to pull the ski boat out of the garage and take it down to a nearby boat launch. The kids were excited to ride in the boat, but Ivan was the only one willing to try and learn to wakeboard. Jordan chose not take a chance at losing his contact lenses in the lake, and the little kids weren't interested in trying. Brian's eight year old son showed off his wake boarding skills first. He was a big kid for eight, quite mature and very strong. Earlier in the summer he had bet his mother that he could pull the ski boat from the middle of the lake into the dock by a rope. She agreed to the bet figuring he couldn't pull it, yet he did. He was an amazing kid.

After Brian's son showed Ivan the finer points of wakeboarding, Ivan took a chance, strapped on the wake board and jumped in. Ivan had snow boarded when he was a little boy, but had never water skied or wake boarded. Ivan tried diligently over the next twenty minutes, but was unable to get up on the board. He would pull up then fall on his face in the water. Between attempts, as he prepared to try again, Ivan's cough became more apparent. I knew this was going to be his one and only chance to ever wakeboard, so I was praying he would make it up. In the back of my mind, I knew in my heart that most likely he would never see another summer. So if he wanted to keep trying, it was fine with me. If it was one of the other kids, I wouldn't have let them even get in the water with such a nasty cough.

When Ivan finally ran out of energy he climbed back in the boat. He was thoroughly chilled and was shaking uncontrollably. I wrapped him in as many towels as I could find. Rich found the hose that blows heat from the engine and we placed it under the towels for added warmth. He continued to shake, his color pale, his coughing now more pronounced. I sat close to him, rubbing his back and attempting to keep the towels from blowing off his thin frame as the boat sped around the lake giving Brian's son one more chance to wake board.

We arrived back at the dock. Ivan was still shaking and pale. He headed into the house to take a bath and try to warm up. I was so glad that he had a chance to try wakeboarding but I could see that the effort had taken a great toll on his body.

Ivan emerged from his hot bath feeling better. That afternoon we ate, fished some more, and sat in the sunshine and relaxed. Jordan and Ivan also worked on their laptop computers. Jordan had just learned over the summer how to take panoramic shots on his digital camera. This was the perfect location. He had taken several still shots during the morning when the mist was hovering over the lake. Now he was attempting to line them up using a special computer program to make a full panoramic portrait of the scene. Both Rich and my dad were professional, or semi-professional photographers, and Jordan was getting a kick out of showing the pro's how it's done. The younger kids and I played board games in the living room next to the two story high rock fireplace. Lenny took Josiah and Sarah out on the lake in the kayaks. We were all engaged in the lake house experience.

After dinner Brian took his kids and started the long commute back to his house. I got the younger kids settled down in their rooms. Jordan was with Josiah in the detached garage apartment waiting for him to fall asleep. All of the kids were tired but happy. Rich had made a fire in the fire place, and I was sitting nearby on the beautiful leather couch. Ivan lay down next to me and plopped his size 12 feet up onto my lap. I began rubbing his feet like I did quite often at home. I loved the closeness I felt with Ivan. He was my big boy, but like a little boy, a part of him still needed to be hugged and held. Though at times he pushed me away, like most teenagers do, more often than not he welcomed me with open arms. The Ivan who used to have a difficult time making eye contact, could now hold eye contact for a long time. At times I felt like we could talk to each other without saying a word, just with our eyes. The saying goes that the eyes are the "window to the soul," and many times I felt I could see into Ivan's soul.

Lenny, Rich, and my parents soon joined Ivan and me near the fire place. We talked over the events of the day, what a magical place this was, and how fortunate we felt to have been invited. Soon Ivan left to join Jordan in the apartment over the garage.

After he left, Rich asked "Is Ivan's cough a cold or the cancer?"

My mind was still trying to chalk it up as a cold that he had caught from Jordan, but I was beginning to wonder. "I don't know." I answered.

Soon our magical weekend at Big Lake was over and we headed home. We all left with hearts full of gratitude for such a wonderful experience. I was still in denial that anything was wrong with Ivan. Despite my preparations, I still hoped a miracle had happened and the cancer had gone away.

Monday morning came too soon after our wonderful weekend away at the lake. Jordan came into my room around 7a.m., a few minutes before he was going to take off for high school. "Ivan's not up yet," he told me. Jordan, Ivan, and Sarah usually rode together. Jordan would drop Sarah off at the middle school before he drove himself and Ivan to the high school. Ivan often would wait until the last minute to get up, grab his back pack, and head out the door. He usually didn't cut the time this close however. I put on a robe and headed to Ivan's room. I knocked quietly then entered. He stirred as I approached him.

"Are you staying home today?" I asked.

"Yes," he replied as he turned over to face me.

"How are your lungs feeling?" I asked.

"I think I have pneumonia. Can you take me to the doctor today?" He questioned.

I realized at that moment that things must be bad. I sure hoped this was pneumonia. Maybe they can just give him an antibiotic and he'll feel better in a few days.

"Would you like to go to Children's or to the clinic?" I asked.

"Not Children's." he stated.

He pretty much had decided after he was told in April that the cancer was back that he would never go back to Seattle Children's Hospital. Except for the quick trip there when he broke his foot, he hadn't had to return. Too many bad memories still lingered there. I assured Ivan that I would make an appointment as soon as the clinic opened at 8 a.m.

I left Ivan and went to say good bye to Jordan and Sarah, and let Jordan know that Ivan was staying home for the day. I let Lenny know that I was concerned that Ivan either had pneumonia or a plural effusion. A plural effusion is where the pleura, or sack around the lung, seeps fluid and causes the lung cavity to fill with fluid causing the lung to collapse. I was aware that this could happen as the tumors in his lungs grew and rubbed on the pleura. My friend with breast cancer had developed this condition towards the end of her life. My mind couldn't deal with the possibility of what that meant for Ivan. I hurried to get dressed and ready for the day, then called the school to let them know of Ivan's absence. I helped Josiah pick out his clothes, get his breakfast, and pack his lunch for school. Kailey and I chatted as I got my breakfast and cleaned the kitchen. I was trying to get everything done so that I could focus on Ivan the rest of the day.

At 8 a.m. I gave Kailey and Josiah a hug and sent them out the door to the bus stop. I placed a call to our pediatrician's office. The first thing in the morning, especially Monday morning, is difficult to get through to the clinic. I tried several times before finally being connected to the scheduler. Our kids' regular pediatrician was unavailable that day, so we were to see a different pediatrician. I had only met this physician one other time at the clinic when I had taken Josiah in for the stomach flu. His only available time was at 4 p.m. Though I was anxious to get Ivan checked out, there was calmness in waiting. I knew from previous conversations with Ivan that he would not allow any extraordinary medical interventions. Oral antibiotics were still on the "ok" list but not much else.

Ivan slept late into the morning. This was common for him even when he was feeling good, so it didn't worry me excessively. I was glad he was able to sleep and not feel so miserable. I spent the day cleaning the house, preparing dinner for that evening, and trying to get ahead of the game. It helped my nerves to be doing something.

Ivan finally woke up, took his shower, and headed out to find something to eat. He seemed run down and continued to have his strange cough. He spent the rest of the day lying on the couch playing the Wii. He didn't look terrible, just a little pale and tired, but not too bad. Maybe this was just a bad cold my mind kept telling me.

I took off to the pediatrician's office with Ivan, leaving Jordan to watch over the rest of the kids. We arrived at the doctor's office. Ivan found a chair as I checked him in. He had his iPod playing so he could tune out the fact that he was actually at the doctor's office. He hated that he saw a pediatrician and was treated at a pediatric hospital. In his mind pediatricians were for kids, and he wasn't a kid anymore. I have to admit, he did look a little out of place there as most of the patients were infants and some grade school kids. Ivan was definitely on the edge of being too old, but this was not the time to be looking for a new doctor.

Shortly after arriving we were called back. The medical assistant asked Ivan to hop on the scale to be weighed. He refused. I gave her a look and a shake of the head that communicated "don't push it." We then headed to the exam room. When the doctor came in I gave him a synopsis of the symptoms that Ivan had been having. He attempted to talk to Ivan, but Ivan refused to answer. Ivan did get on the exam table but then he kept his head down and eyes looking at the floor, elbows on his knees. The pediatrician did his physical exam. He commented that he could not hear much air movement from the right lung. He told Ivan that he needed a chest x-ray and then left the room. As soon as the doctor left Ivan said "I'm not going to have an x-ray." I spent the next couple minutes trying to convince him that it was needed to see if it was pneumonia or something else. He adamantly refused. When the medical assistant came in to take him for the x-ray, I pulled her out of the room and went to speak with the doctor. I told him that Ivan was refusing to have an x-ray. At this point, I felt Ivan needed control more than the x-ray. I also knew that Ivan was stubborn enough that unless we sedated him and carried him to the machine, he wouldn't go anyways. The doctor agreed to put him on antibiotics in case this was pneumonia instead of cancer. We all knew that this was most likely was not the virus that Jordan had. We scheduled another appointment at the end of the week for Ivan to be checked by our regular doctor.

During the week, prior to seeing our regular pediatrician, I was trying to convince myself that he was getting better.

"Take a breath" I listened to his lungs. When I was listening to the left side everything sounded clear and normal. I moved my stethoscope to his right side.

"Take a breath." I could hear nothing. "Are you holding your breath?" I asked, thinking Ivan was playing one of his tricks on me.

"No." Ivan replied.

After several attempts I could tell he was breathing but there was no air moving into his right lung. I knew then that this wasn't pneumonia.

The following Friday I took Ivan back to see our regular pediatrician. He listened to his lungs and confirmed there was no air moving on his right side. Again the doctor asked Ivan to have a chest x-ray. Ivan refused. The pediatrician gently explained that either the tumor had grown across a main bronchus, or he had a pleural effusion and the right lung was full of fluid. Either way his right lung was no longer functioning. He explained to Ivan that if it was a pleural effusion, the fluid could be tapped off which would give him some relief for a while. Without an x-ray he was unable to tell what was going on. Ivan remained quiet, not asking questions. This was altogether different. After Monday's appointment we still had a glimmer of hope that the antibiotics would fix the problem. We now knew that this was the beginning of the end. I left the pediatricians office numb. When I asked Ivan how he was doing he was always nonchalant.

"Are you scared? Angry?" I'd ask.

"No." was always the reply. He acted like it was just any other day.

I often felt scared, sad, and angry. It often felt like Ivan and I were on this roller coaster ride together, yet alone. Others could check in and out of the pain. For us, it wasn't a choice, Ivan and I had to go to the appointments and hear the dreadful news. As his mom, it was my job, and I wouldn't want it any other way. I just wished someone else would accompany us. I wasn't strong enough to bear this grief alone. Of course Lenny had to work and the kids had school. It was difficult for Seneca to be involved while trying to support himself financially. I also felt that emotionally it was difficult for Seneca to see Ivan's health deteriorate. Seneca was a deep soul and he was losing the closest family member that he had. I knew his absence was not an indicator of his lack of care, but his inability to cope with the situation. I felt Ivan was stronger than I, but I didn't want him to have to support me emotionally. Besides he would just say "Get over it" or call me a "whiner" with a smirk when I'd show any sadness.

When we returned home I slipped into my room to call his Nurse Practitioner, Sue. I told her what had happened and that I felt it was time to get hospice involved. I knew that if things got worse Ivan would not go to the hospital and I needed the tools like oxygen and different medications here to help him. I had no idea how long he had left. Days, weeks, months, all I knew is that I didn't want to do it without hospice.

During the time that I cared for my grandfather and my friend with breast cancer, I'd learned how valuable hospice was. The two of them died at our home, 10 days apart. Both of them were bedridden and in the dying process for 3-4 months. I could not have taken care of them without the guidance and help of hospice. Sue said that she would make the referral the following week. I was sure hoping Ivan would not continue to decline rapidly over the weekend.

I also called to let Seneca know what was going on with his brother. We made plans for him to come up from Seattle a few days later. Since the adoption in June, Seneca had been coming around much more frequently. During those visits he began to share with me some of the struggles he had been dealing with since Ivan moved into our home. Not only had he felt like we had taken his brother from him, he'd also lost his place to live when they left the Ronald McDonald House. He was essentially homeless for the first few months after Ivan moved in with us. The picture of what Seneca had been going through was becoming clearer. Often he was trying to find a new place to stay with no place to store his belongings. He moved between friends houses, and often slept at the tattoo shop after he would close it up for the night just to be able to sleep indoors. It now made sense why he would never pick up his belongings from the Ronald McDonald house. He had no place to store them. He had been very angry with us, and had no desire to form any relationships here. Beyond that he had fallen into a deep depression, feeling like he had lost his brother again. His absence for all those months finally started to make sense.

Seneca remained Ivan's favorite person. They had a connection and love for each other that was unquestionable. I felt completely loved by Ivan, but I also knew that Ivan was happiest when Seneca was with him. I had also developed a deep caring for Seneca. I worried about him almost as much as I did Ivan. Ivan was Seneca's closest relative. Loosing Ivan would be beyond devastating for him. I had tried my hardest to prove to Seneca that we cared about him, and that we wanted him here as much as he could find the time to be with us. We wanted to be like family to him. I think he was starting to almost believe that.

Over the weekend Ivan's coughing became noticeably worse. Anytime he moved or would lie flat he would go into a coughing fit. I was worried about him and wanted to be with him all the time. I know my hovering drove him nuts at times but at other times he wanted me near. When the kids were gone to school he'd often hang out with me. He'd lie on the couch and flop his feet in my lap for another foot rub, or I'd rub his head until he'd fall asleep. When I was doing something for him I felt better. If he was just lying there coughing, it broke my heart.

Several days after Sue made the referral to hospice, the nurse came out to do the intake and get him started. The night before they were to come I told Ivan. Ivan was upset that I had requested hospice. He was sure that we could do it together and didn't need any other nurses. I explained that he may need oxygen and pain meds to help him stay at home. He assured me that he wouldn't use the oxygen or take the pain meds. I expressed to him that he may change his mind and I wanted them to be on hand if he did. He said he would refuse any medical treatments. I told him that he may not need or want anyone else, but I wanted the assistance. I tried to explain it like childbirth. Some people give birth in a hospital with a lot of medical intervention, and others have a home birth with a midwife and very little medical care. But it isn't cool to just go squat behind a tree and give birth. We are doing it like the home birth I explained, we needed a little help. I told him that I would try to not have the nurses touch him or even talk to him much, but they are going to be available to me. He agreed with that plan.

When the nurse came I sat and spoke with her out of earshot of Ivan. She understood that Ivan was intensely unhappy with hospice being involved and she was accommodating to him. Hospice nurses usually do a thorough exam on their first visit. Our nurse agreed to forgo the exam and only asked him a couple questions, then left him alone. I know Ivan appreciated that the nurse respected him enough to give him his space and didn't force him to undergo an exam. She did order the oxygen and pain medications, along with all the other medications that help someone who is dying. As the meds and equipment were delivered, I'd mention it to

Ivan, then put the equipment out of sight.

Seneca made it out the evening after the hospice nurse was at our house. He and Ivan asked if I could drop them off at the mall to get Ivan's computer fixed. I was reluctant because I wasn't sure how Ivan would be able to handle it, but I also knew that if it was important to Ivan, I should try to let him go. About an hour after I dropped them off I got a text to come pick them up. As they approached the car I could tell Ivan was physically exhausted. He was coughing and breathing hard, he looked pale. Ivan stated that he had a headache. It was difficult to see him looking so bad. I wondered if this was Ivan's last trip to the mall or perhaps anywhere.

We got home and got Ivan comfortable. I gave Seneca a ride back down to his apartment. On the ride I asked Seneca if he would consider moving in with us. I knew from caring for my Grandfather and my friend Joyce, that nursing someone who was in the process of dying was a full time job for several people. I had cared for the two of them with some help from an aide, along with my parents and hospice guiding me, but it had been extremely difficult for me to do it all. Even though Ivan was just one person, I knew I would need someone to help me. Lenny was working and would be needed to tend to the kids while my attention was on Ivan's care. Besides me, I knew the only person Ivan would feel comfortable receiving help from was his brother. Beyond the assistance I needed to care for Ivan, was the knowledge that the brothers needed to be together during this time. Seneca needed to be with a family during and after Ivan's death, and I needed him also. Even though we adopted Ivan and not Seneca, in my heart we had adopted both of them. Seneca still seemed somewhat reserved and a bit uncomfortable at our house, but I hoped if he lived here, that would fade away.

Away from the house, usually when I'd drive him home, we would have long talks about life, death, religion, and his and Ivan's childhood...all sorts of meaningful conversations. Seneca had a deep soul and I very much appreciated that in him. I think I've scared some people away by talking about topics that are deep, when they feel more comfortable sticking to surface talk. Seneca said he would think about moving in.

A few months earlier he had moved in with a friend and was splitting the rent with him. Seneca had recently become unemployed when the tattoo and piercing shop he had been working at closed. I was worried about Seneca. He was struggling financially, along with dealing with his brother's illness. Seneca was also concerned for his roommate, as he had committed to pay half the rent. He was in the process of trying to find another job to be able to pay his share. He was carrying a huge load.

Over the next couple of weeks Seneca would spend a day or two with us and then return to his apartment. We had moved Jordan and Josiah back together in one room to make a place for Seneca to sleep when he'd spend the night. He seemed uncomfortable about making food for himself while he was here. Similar to when Ivan first moved in, I encouraged him to just make himself at home and eat whatever he wanted, but this was difficult for him. We were used to having new foster kids and other people staying in our house, rummaging through our cupboards and refrigerator. We explained to him that it didn't bother us.

Ivan was still able to move about the house, though it would trigger long coughing jags. It was getting difficult for him to lie flat in his bed. At night I'd hear him coughing uncontrollably, sometimes for hours.

I'd go in and check on him which at times annoyed him. He'd say "I'm just coughing." Occasionally I'd lay across the foot of his bed because I was so worried about him. The incessant coughing rattled me and I would have images of finding him dead in the morning.

I knew that he would probably do better in a hospital bed with the head elevated, but that was out of the question. Instead, I put a large floor pillow under the head of his mattress to elevate it a little, which unfortunately didn't seem to give him much relief.

One day while we were alone I gently asked him. "Do you worry about dying? Does it make you afraid?" He was so calm about the whole topic. He said he wasn't afraid and he didn't worry. Again he encouraged me to "Get over it." After our conversation he was quite affectionate and sat near me playing with my hands. I wasn't sure if he was trying to comfort me or himself.

CHAPTER 10

Ivan's 17th birthday came on October 14th. I invited all the people that had become close to Ivan over the 14 months that he had been with our family. Over 25 people came, including his grandma and his cousin from California. Just a couple of years earlier he felt like he had been thrown away, with no family or friends who cared about him. Now he was surrounded by people who loved him deeply. It did my heart good to see all the love being poured out on him. We all knew this was Ivan's last birthday, which made the grief overwhelming. Ivan did well hiding how sick he really was at the party. He'd occasionally escape to his bedroom to lie down for a while, or go and cough violently only to return a few minutes later and act as healthy as he could. I also knew that this was most likely the last time many of these friends and family would get to spend time with Ivan. We made it as festive as possible despite the circumstances.

Just prior to Ivan's 17th birthday, Seneca made the move into our house. I was so grateful. I felt it would be better for all of us to be together, and it was. Seneca started applying for work at our nearby mall and soon got a job. The job, stocking merchandise at a retail store, had odd hours. He needed to be to work very early in the morning before the buses ran. I began driving him each morning, around 5 a.m. This worked for a while, but within a few weeks of him taking the job, Ivan became weaker. I begged Seneca to stop working so he could be available to help. I could tell all the stress on Seneca was taking its toll. It was difficult for him to work while worrying about how his brother was doing at home. It was also difficult for me to get enough rest. Seneca agreed to stop working, which made life much easier for all of us.

As the days went by and Ivan's health declined, he'd walk around less and cough more. Pain started becoming more of an issue in his back, sides, and right shoulder. He refused the morphine that the hospice had ordered, but would occasionally take Tylenol. I could tell that the Tylenol didn't touch the pain.

Ivan had always loved backrubs. As the pain increased, he found that they helped ease the pain and allowed him to relax. For weeks, Ivan relied on them instead of narcotic pain meds. But just as I thought, the pain soon became unbearable. I was so relieved we had the Morphine already in the house and didn't have to wait a day or two for it to be delivered. When he finally relented and agreed to take the stronger pain medication it did give him relief.

By the beginning of November, it was getting very difficult for Ivan to walk around the house. He would have to hold onto the counter in the kitchen, and the furniture in the living room as he made his way to and from his room. He was no longer able to sleep lying down. In the rec. room a chair and a half that reclined became Ivan's bed, and the rec. room his bedroom. It functioned like a hospital bed for Ivan, without having him be in a real hospital bed which satisfied him.

All along as Ivan was getting increasingly more ill, I was still taking care of my elderly grandmother, in addition to our other 5 children. It became too much for me to manage. We made arrangements for Grandma Rose to go spend time with my aunt until things settled down.

The kids continued to interact with Ivan. They watched television and played video games with him when he was up to it. However, now things were drastically changing. They all loved him deeply and wanted to continue to be with him, but their time together needed to be limited. He was just too tired to keep up with their energy.

Most of my emotional and physical energy was now going towards Ivan at this point. I felt bad for the other kids and Lenny, but I also knew this was just a short season of time. Many of our friends and relatives stepped up and would take the kids on the weekends to their houses. It got them out of the house and tried to let them have some normalcy and fun. I knew this was helpful to them in many ways, yet some of the kids would have rather stayed home and just sat quietly with

Ivan. He was their brother and they hurt terribly watching him suffer.

Lenny would work all day and then come home to take over all the household duties that were usually mine. He worked double time since I could no longer keep up with managing the household chores. We were blessed when multiple people began bringing us meals. It was so helpful not having to worry about fixing dinner a few days a week. Besides not having to cook a meal, it made us feel that people cared about our family and what we were all going through.

The old depressed, shut down, introverted Ivan was long gone, even in his dying the fun and loving teenager was still there. While he was quite weak and sick, Ivan still never lost his ability to have a little bit of fun. Before Seneca stopped working at the mall he had picked up a package of jelly beans that were disgusting flavors like dirt, dish soap, vomit and earwax. When his unsuspecting sibling or visitors would stop by to visit him, he'd offer them a colorful jelly bean. Unaware of what they were about to eat, his guests would get a nasty surprise. Ivan would get a quick laugh watching their reactions. Though his body was failing him, his spirit was strong. His fun personality was still present. It helped lighten the mood of an otherwise very depressing situation.

Our youth pastor from church, Phil, had invested a lot into Ivan over the past several months. He had taken him places when he was well and then came to visit him at the house once he had become ill. One time when Pastor Phil stopped by, Ivan was getting very weak. He would stand up only a few times a day and could only walk a couple steps. They talked for a bit and watched a show together. Ivan was dozing in and out. Phil quietly said goodbye and begun to sneak out. As he was walking towards the door, I noticed Ivan trying to stand up on his weak and wobbly legs. I instinctively knew that Ivan had stood to give Phil a hug. I called to Phil who turned and came back to embrace Ivan. The little energy that Ivan had left was spent to express his love. The pastor who was always giving to others left with a gift and tears in his eyes.

By mid-November, Ivan got to the point that he was requiring round the clock pain medications. Seneca and I would take turns sleeping on the couch next to him, or one of us would sleep on the floor and the other on the couch so that we could care for him in the night.

Several days in a row around 5 a.m. while I was dozing on the couch, I would hear Ivan attempting to stand up. He would get himself to a standing position, take a couple steps, and stand next to me. The first time I had no idea what was happening. It was Ivan requesting a hug and giving me a gift of his love. In that hug he was saying "thank you" and "I love you" without uttering a word. I'd stand and hug him and then he would climb into his chair and fall back asleep. For multiple days he did this until he could no longer come to a standing position on his own.

The pain and shortness of breath were always present. One evening I had stepped into the living room to spend some time with the rest of the family, Seneca was hanging out with Ivan in the rec. room. All of a sudden Seneca came rushing into where I was and said "We need the oxygen now!" I ran to the rec. room as Ivan sat gasping for air, shaking, and in a complete sweat. Seneca had gone to get the oxygen and I sat there holding my boy as he gasped with a panicked look in his eyes. We were quickly able to get the oxygen on him and he settled down. The look of panic in his eyes is an image that will forever be burned in my memory.

Because of Ivan's aversion to anything hospital or medical, he never allowed us to put the oxygen cannula on him. He would just hold the end of the tube in front of his face to breath the oxygen. This made it tricky as he would fade in and out of sleep and drop the oxygen tubing. It was a full time job for Seneca and me to keep repositioning the oxygen tubing near his face. I tried to convince him of the benefits of wearing the oxygen cannula but he remained stubborn even in his frail health.

From mid-November on he was no longer able to sleep reclined in the chair. He would sleep nearly sitting straight up with pillows propping his head, or he would flop over a stack of pillows on the side of the chair. It looked very uncomfortable. Between the shortness of breath and the pain, Ivan had a difficult time sleeping for more than a couple hours. Seneca and I were up with him whenever he was awake. We would take turns kneeling in front of him as he wrapped his arms around our shoulders in an attempt to be able to breathe easier. We would try to catch naps, but all three of us became very weary and sleep deprived.

One night after we all had been awake for what seemed like days on end, we had come to a point of utter exhaustion. I crawled into the chair with Ivan and began to rub his back and head. He relaxed and finally fell asleep in my arms. I could feel his warm sleeping body breathing and I cherished this moment. I knew that all too soon I would not have him to love and hold. All three of us fell sound asleep, and slept for five hours. That was the longest stretch of sleep any of us got in a couple of weeks. That stretch of sleep with Ivan wrapped in my arms felt like a precious gift from God. We all woke up feeling a bit better. I loved this boy so much. The thought of him no longer being present would send me into tears while he slept. At times, with Ivan sleeping next to us, Seneca and I would sob quietly together. The pain would overwhelm us.

Several times during Ivan's last couple weeks he would start talking about seeing things or people. He said he was seeing sparkling diamonds at one point.

One time he asked "Who are those two people?"

I asked him "What people?"

Then he said "The two chicks in white."

189

I replied "Maybe they are angels."

To which Seneca asked "Are they hot?"

Ivan smirked, but then drifted back off to sleep. Many people would say it was the pain meds causing him to hallucinate. I'd rather think he was getting glimpses of heaven.

Ivan had always done better with non-verbal communication, verbal I love you's made him uncomfortable. So I decided to write him a letter to express all that was in my heart for him.

Ivan,

I love you! I know all the "sappy," "mushy," love stuff makes you feel uncomfortable so I don't say it too often. But I want you to know for sure how much you are loved. I wish you had many more years on this earth to experience that love in your life, but that looks like it won't be the case. I've prayed and begged God for a miracle for you, hoping you'd beat the odds with this type of cancer. The only thing I can hold onto is that this life is just the beginning, there is still eternity. Eternity is our hope, life doesn't end when this earthly life is done. You know I have told you before how I think about how birth and death are the same in so many ways. Before a baby is born he only knows what he/she has experienced in the womb, which is very limited. If you tried to explain the world to that unborn baby it would not make any sense. I believe death is like birth only we are "birthed" into heaven. Heaven is unexplainable to our human minds, but it is real and it is good. From what I've read about people who have had near death experiences it is so good that they are reluctant to even come back to this earth. The peace, love, and joy that they experience is so real they don't want to leave it. I believe that they are experiencing God's heart for them when they feel that overwhelming love and peace. I know you made a commitment to God when you were in Montana, and you've told me that you never "felt" like anything happened. I wish you could have tangibly felt God's love for you on earth. You will just have to believe that he absolutely loves you and he did hear your prayer. I believe he sent you to our family and maybe that prayer was what started things (we will never know). I hope you can see the love our family, friends, Phil M, Phil P,

Susan, etc. have given to you is God loving you through us. He maybe thought you needed love with skin on instead of just a feeling that God loves you. My prayer and hope now is that you will let us comfort and love you through this process, then hand you over to someone (God) that loves you more than Seneca or I or anyone could ever love you. Then some day we will be reunited in a place where there will be no more pain or suffering. It will be a place that we cannot imagine this side, but is totally awesome. That is what I hold on to as I have to let go of you for now.

Love, Hugs, and Foot rubs

Mom(i.e.Cindy)

On November 25th, the Sunday after Thanksgiving, Ivan had a restless night. Seneca and I had been giving him oral pain meds every couple of hours through the night. As soon as he would awaken we would try to get a med in him before he would start hurting. Seneca was asleep on the floor. I heard Ivan starting to move around. I got up quickly to get his medication since it had been three hours since his last dose. I tried to give it to him but he refused. He was having a difficult time with his breathing, so I kneeled in front of him so he could wrap his arms around me to help with his breathing. I held him as he struggled for air. Seneca heard us moving around and woke. He sat there on the floor briefly trying to wake up. Ivan in a whisper said "Hug" to Seneca. Seneca crawled over and took over holding Ivan. The brothers held each other for several minutes, then Seneca laid him back into the chair as we both wrapped ourselves around him. Ivan's breathing changed and I knew what it meant. I whispered to Seneca that this was the end. We sat there holding him and telling him how much we loved him, how much we would miss him, and that it was ok to go. My precious boy took his last breath enveloped in love, the love that he deserved, a love that felt elusive to him for so many years of his life.

In his own way of communicating, Ivan showed that his words were not needed to convey his unquestionable love. He spoke with his eyes, his touch, and his heart. I heard him, and he changed my world forever.

I got to be the mom that Ivan loved

I got to be the mom who loved Ivan.

I got to be the one who watched him come out of his shell.

I got to see the introvert turn into the extrovert that he was created to be.

I got to be the recipient of Ivan's pranks and random silliness.

I got to be the mom who held him as he grieved over the pain of his past.

When his strength was failing, I'm the mom he hugged to make sure I knew how much he loved me.

I got to be the mom who held and comforted him while he was dying.

I got to be the mom that shared with him the hope of eternity and how much God loved him.

I got to be the mom who held his face in my hands as he took his last breath.

I got to be the mom that Ivan loved.

Cindy Locke

ABOUT THE AUTHOR

Cindy Locke began working with children as a rehabilitation nurse at Seattle Children's Hospital. Seeing children go through the hospital with little or no family support compelled her to become a foster parent. Along with her husband Lenny, Cindy has been a foster parent for over 25 years. Together they have parented more than 30 foster children, many with disabilities and life threatening medical conditions. She is the mother of three adopted and three biological children. Cindy continues to do foster care along with volunteering at Safe Place, a 72 hour shelter for children removed in emergency situations.

Made in the USA
San Bernardino, CA
01 April 2016